CLINICAL EXERCISE TESTING

NORMAN L. JONES, M.D. (Lond.), F.R.C.P. (Lond.) F.R.C.P. (C.)

Professor of Medicine
McMaster University, Hamilton

E. J. MORAN CAMPBELL, M.D. (Lond.), Ph.D. (Lond.), F.R.C.P. (Lond.), F.R.C.P. (C.)

McLaughlin Professor of Medicine and
Chairman, Department of Medicine
McMaster University, Hamilton

RICHARD H. T. EDWARDS, B.Sc., Ph.D. (Lond.), M.B., M.R.C.P. (Lond.)

Lecturer, Department of Medicine
Royal Postgraduate Medical School, and
Honorary Consultant Physician,
Hammersmith Hospital, London

DENIS G. ROBERTSON, F.R.A.C.P.

Physician and Chairman of Section of Thoracic Medicine,
Alfred Hospital, Melbourne;
Formerly Lecturer, Department of Medicine,
McMaster University, Hamilton

W. B. SAUNDERS COMPANY
Philadelphia, London, Toronto

W. B. Saunders Company: West Washington Square
Philadelphia, PA 19105

1 St. Anne's Road
Eastbourne, East Sussex BN21 3UN, England

1 Goldthorne Avenue
Toronto, Ontario M8Z 5T9, Canada

Library of Congress Cataloging in Publication Data

Main entry under title:

Clinical exercise testing.

Includes index.

1. Exercise tests.   I. Jones, Norman Longden. [DNLM:
   1. Exercise test.   2. Exertion. WE103 C641]

RC71.8.C58   616.07'54   74–25477

ISBN 0–7216–5226–3

Clinical Exercise Testing   ISBN   0-7216-5226-3

Last digit is the print number: 9   8   7   6   5   4   3

Preface

This is a practical book aimed at two groups of readers; clinicians who wish to know something of the value, indications, and interpretation of exercise tests; and clinicians and clinical physiologists who have responsibility for cardiorespiratory investigation laboratories, who are presently making little use of exercise testing but wish to do so, or who are practicing exercise testing and wish to know our approach and obtain a source of background information.

A number of books about exercise have appeared recently, but most are more concerned with the physiology of athletic performance than with clinical physiology. Over the last decade, first at the Royal Postgraduate Medical School and then at the institutions where we now work, we have evolved a general approach to exercise testing which we have found useful in clinical investigation.

We have deliberately restricted the reviews of physiology and pathophysiology to simple accounts with reference to reviews of the literature. In addition, we have described the procedures we use with only limited reference to alternative methods; there are others, but these alternatives must be judged with regard to their reliability and their applicability to a wide range of clinical situations. Studying patients during exercise presents technical problems whose subtleties are not obvious; we hope that our experience will benefit others.

Our approach to exercise testing is integrative in the sense of Barcroft's remark, "It seems impossible to escape from the conception that the adaptation to exercise is an integration of a large number of factors, no one of which would alter sufficiently to be completely effective."

Many mechanisms come into play in exercise, and the ability to work efficiently depends not only on their integrity but also on their integration. Exercise may be limited by malfunction of any factor, but the body is capable of remarkable adaptation to a weak link in the chain. Increasing exercise will stress such an adaptation to the limit, often leading to a break in the chain at a point remote from the weak link that provided the first strain. For this reason, as many as possible of these mechanisms should be explored fully at several increasing loads; measurements at a single work rate may be less informative, because the test will not be an equal stress for all patients and may fail to reveal the mechanisms which limit adaptation to an increasing power output.

Exercise testing should be considered an extension of the clinical examination. In engineering it is axiomatic that testing under load is a necessary step in the assessment of any machine. Why, therefore, has testing of the human machine been so little practiced until recently and is still often approached in a superficial manner? The answer may lie in the seeming complexity of techniques and physiological processes, and in a vague fear of risk. Mainly for these reasons we have tried to develop techniques which are simple and free of risk. Simple techniques critically applied can often obviate the need for more complex studies; the information gained from a bloodless study may be all that is required for the adequate assessment of the patient.

At first sight, exercise testing would seem to be risky, and it is undeniable that exercise may be hazardous in some conditions. However, we would challenge the view that questioning a patient about the severity of exercise he can undertake, unobserved and uncontrolled, is safer than close observation of his controlled performance supplemented by objective measurements. Furthermore, we would challenge the practice of allowing some patients, for example those with ischemic heart disease, to follow a daily routine of activity in occupation or sport, with historical data and observations at rest as the only guides to cardiac function.

We hope that the reader will be able to judge the importance of exercise testing, learn how to perform the tests reliably, and become familiar with the interpretation of results to obtain maximal information from them.

Because we hope to attract readers with a wide range of experience, the book falls into two parts. The first (Chaps. 1–3) consists of a general introduction to exercise testing, the physiology of exercise, the factors influencing the choice of techniques, and a description of the techniques we have found most helpful. The second part (Chaps. 4–12) deals with detailed questions of equipment, procedure, and interpretation of results. Some technical graphs and tables appear as an appendix.

N. L. JONES

Acknowledgements

This book was conceived almost a decade ago at the Royal Postgraduate Medical School; during its lengthy gestation we have drawn on the experience and critical comments of many colleagues who worked with us at the School, and later at the institutions where we now work. Several made original contributions to its development or its writing; Dr. Ross McHardy provided much of the early momentum to the use of rebreathing for the measurement of mixed venous PCO_2 in bloodless exercise tests and in the analysis of results; Dr. Simon Godfrey contributed his experience gained in exercise testing of children, and also improved the manuscript during successive drafts; Mr. Jim Kane, Mr. Ted Davies and Mr. Ray Fautley applied their expertise to the development of equipment, and Mr. Monte Smith to the computer applications. To Dr. Charles Fletcher and Sir John McMichael we extend our gratitude for their encouragement and forbearance, and to Dr. John West, Dr. John Sutton, Dr. Arnold Naimark, and Dr. Tony Rebuck for many discussions on topics of mutual interest. We have learned much from many friends in Scandinavia, Great Britain, and Canada and hope we have acknowledged our debt to them in various parts of the book.

Our work has been supported generously by grants from the Medical Research Councils of Great Britain and Canada, the Chest and Heart Association, the Wates Foundation, and the Ontario Thoracic Society. Dr. John Wicks read the manuscript with great care. At all stages in the production we have been indebted to Sylvia Skomorowski, who typed successive drafts with great speed and accuracy. Finally it is a pleasure to acknowledge the help of Mr. Brian Decker and his colleagues at Saunders in bringing the book to its publication.

Contents

Chapter One

AN INTRODUCTION TO EXERCISE TESTING

There are a number of points to be made at the outset, some of which are developed in more depth elsewhere but which we believe should be borne in mind from the beginning.

WHY USE EXERCISE TESTING?

Disease of an organ or system reduces its reserve capacity — its capacity to respond to increasing demands. Most organs have a large reserve, and clinical manifestations occur only when their capacity is greatly reduced. Thus the relationship between a clinical symptom and the severity of the underlying function derangement is nonlinear. This is one of the reasons why an assessment of exercise tolerance based on the patient's history is very insensitive. Symptomatic limitation of exercise tolerance depends on the function of the whole organism, including the subjective response to stress. Let us now examine these points in greater detail.

LIMITATIONS OF THE ASSESSMENT OF EXERCISE TOLERANCE BY QUESTIONING

The reserve physiological capacity of the circulatory and respiratory systems is such that it is possible to lose much of this capacity before the demands of daily living become compromised. Once this loss has occurred, major changes in exercise tolerance may result,

1

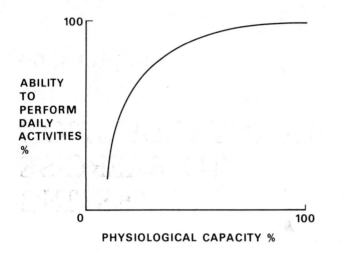

Figure 1-1

with only small changes in the capacity of the primarily affected organ or system.

These two concepts are expressed diagrammatically in Figure 1-1, in which the ordinate clearly depends upon the individual, his activities, and his culture but might extend to walking quickly, cycling or swimming, or to competitive athletics. On the abscissa, physiological capacity represents the maximum capacity to breathe, to transfer oxygen in the lungs, to increase cardiac output, to transport oxygen by the blood, to perfuse the active muscle, and so on. Whatever the detailed variations in the axes, the general shape is certainly convex upwards with a flat upper part in which major changes in the functional capacity of organs cause few symptoms unless strenuous exercise is taken, and a lower steeper part in which major changes in symptoms may signify relatively little change in the function of the affected organ.

CLINICAL ASSESSMENT OF EXERCISE TOLERANCE

Exercise Tolerance as Assessed Clinically Depends on the Whole Organism

The effect of limitation of a physiological process on exercise tolerance depends not only on its severity but also upon the other processes concerned in exercise; these may mask or aggravate the effects of the main abnormality and may determine symptoms during exercise and their severity. Thus limitation of the ability to transfer oxygen in the lungs may be disguised by an increase in breathing; limitation of the ability to increase cardiac output may be disguised by a greater extraction of oxygen from blood and by diversion of blood from nonexercising tissues.

An important practical corollary to the physiological truism stated above is that clinical improvement may depend on attention to other mechanisms in addition to that primarily affected by disease. There is no need to labor the point that symptoms arising from the same limitation vary in different subjects and in the same subject at different times depending upon many factors.

Exercise Performance as Assessed Clinically Is an "Unsteady State" Affair

Looked at broadly, an examination of exercise performance might range from studies of single motor unit contractions, through maximal brief muscle contraction and isometric power of several muscle groups, to dynamic exercise of long duration. However, in this book we are concerned with dynamic exercise involving large muscle groups for at least several minutes and requiring complex energy supply mechanisms. Many activities in everyday life are brief, particularly those involving a high output of power and in which many of these mechanisms do not adapt fully during the time of the exercise; in this sense the mechanisms never reach the "steady state" beloved of exercise physiologists. The standard clinical questions, "How far can you walk?" or "How many stairs can you climb?", seek information regarding maximal performance in what is usually "un-steady state" exercise. Consider stair-climbing: the power output achieved in climbing is usually beyond the ability of the respiratory and circulatory systems to sustain in a "steady state," though we know that one or two flights can be climbed without even taking a breath. The answer to the common clinical question "How many stairs can you climb without getting short of breath?" must lie somewhere between 30 and 120 stairs or two to six domestic flights. Less than this can be accomplished without employing the heart or lungs, and more is within the compass of an athlete only. Of course, this argument is a caricature. Although we may climb 30 stairs at a rate in excess of our ability to meet the energy demands, we do not have to meet the cost immediately; we "buy now and pay later." Patients often esti-mate the cost of exercise from their experience of the difficulty they have in paying the bill later, when the severity of dyspnea indicates how close they are to the limit of their ability to repay. Nevertheless, the evaluation of exercise tolerance by questioning alone leaves much to be desired; it becomes increasingly unrealistic as limitation becomes increasingly severe and even minor activity becomes limited by the patient's willingness to tolerate distress (Campbell, 1967).

Having made these points we do not wish to imply that testing patients during exercise necessarily is superior to an assessment based on their stated ability to perform certain activities; the two are complementary, the information of each being directed towards different ends. Exercise testing is directed towards measurement of individual components of the system; the symptoms experienced by a patient when he performs a certain activity depend on the way the whole person responds to the environment.

The question of unsteady versus steady state exercise will arise again when the design of exercise testing protocols is considered. At this juncture we would make two points only. First, as long as dynamic exercise at several power outputs is studied, there is no need to adhere slavishly to the steady state, particularly if variables are related to each other rather than to an absolute power output. Secondly, we do not deny that a steady state is required for certain calculations to be made; however, a completely steady state in all mechanisms is an unattainable goal—mechanisms need only be steady enough to allow the valid application of measurements made during the test.

PRELIMINARY CONSIDERATIONS IN EXERCISE TESTING

How May Exercise Testing Be Most Effectively Used?

Exercise testing must examine all component systems and the integration and interaction between them. An exercise test should reveal not only the primary malfunction but also should demonstrate whether other mechanisms are hiding, disguising, or aggravating the primary defect. This provides the added benefit that the performance of the systems can be examined in relation to each other rather than in relation to established normal standards alone. To accomplish this requires testing at several work rates. Exercise testing based upon the use of a single standard level of exercise may add little to studies made at rest, for it may represent no stress for one patient while being too high for another.

Exercise Testing Should be "Cost Effective"

Recently there has been much concern regarding the cost of patient investigation in relation to its value in diagnosis or treatment.

Few investigations have been realistically assessed in this way, and indeed such an assessment often may be impossible. However, the responsibility should not be shirked, and as a first step we feel that the desired information should be provided with the least cost. Unfortunately, technical innovation has led to the development of complex and expensive procedures, which are used in many cardiorespiratory laboratories. Although exercise testing may be added to these procedures, their complexity may make it difficult to obtain simpler information which is more applicable to the functional assessment of the patient. Hence the "cost" of this approach is compounded.

A major motive underlying our work has been to extend the benefit and to lessen the cost of simple noninvasive tests so that we can apply the simplest and least invasive technique that will give the required information. Our object is to describe the available choices for those wishing to use exercise testing as part of clinical investigation.

Exercise Testing Is a Clinical Procedure

"Routine" exercise tests are valuable, and it is certainly necessary to have a routine, but a test is more informative if addressed to a particular clinical problem and conducted in such a way as to yield a specific answer.

If exercise is used as part of the assessment of certain clinical problems, it soon becomes clear that it is of greater value in early than in advanced disease. In a patient who is so limited as to be capable of very little exercise, the results are largely predictable and may add little to the clinical examination, apart from an objective assessment of symptoms.

Finally, a change in a simple measurement repeated over a period of time is often more helpful than a more complicated measurement made once in the course of the patient's illness. If assessment is based on simple techniques, it is possible to study patients more frequently.

It is a common practice in pulmonary function testing to supply the referring clinician with a battery of numbers (often expressed as "percentage of normal") followed by an expert interpretation that is usually descriptive, often redundant, and rarely as clinically useful as it ought to be. We recognize the reasons for this state of affairs but wish to escape and certainly not to encourage it.

The information we aim to provide does not depend upon advanced theory. We seek to answer such simple questions as, "How much air does this patient breathe?"; "How much blood does his heart pump?"; "Is he limited more by his ability to breathe or to pump blood?"; "Is the volume of air he is breathing or blood he is pumping, more or less than it should be or used to be, when stressed by exercise?". We hope this book will provide clinicians with the information necessary to answer such questions from measurements made during exercise.

WHAT IS A "NORMAL" RESPONSE TO EXERCISE?

The problem of establishing normal standards will emerge frequently in this book, as it does in practice. It might appear to be a question that would be settled easily by population studies carried out by those who conduct exercise tests and who then use the data to interpret their results. However, the problem is in fact rather more difficult and, paradoxically, the solution easier than this simple approach would indicate. The definition of a "normal" population is a complex task. The exercise performance of most people in the Western world can be improved by regular exercise. One might, therefore, take for normal values the results of studies of those who take exercise regularly, but such standards might not be easy to apply to the results of a test performed in a patient who has not taken any exercise for years. Even if results from an appropriate population are available, there remains the problem of defining limits, with the attendant risks of including false positives and false negatives. Fortunately, the situation becomes less troublesome with increasing familiarity as the clinician uses the numerical values to complement other clinical investigations and finds that more information is obtained from the relationship between variables rather than from the value of each considered by itself. Thus we have done our best to indicate "normal" values, but we hope that these will be used for orientation rather than as rigid criteria for the diagnosis of abnormality.

INDICATIONS FOR EXERCISE TESTING

A brief review of the clinical uses of exercise testing underlines some of the major objectives of the book. We gain better appreciation of the patient's symptoms, the severity of impaired function, and the diagnosis.

Objective Assessment of Symptoms

The patient is often referred because exercise performance is limited by certain symptoms. An exercise test should quantify the limitation objectively, and clarify the patient's description by assessing his reaction at the time of the test.

Assessment of Impaired Function

Quantitative information can be obtained regarding the following systems and processes: ventilation and pulmonary gas exchange; central and peripheral circulation; blood gas transport; and peripheral gas exchange and metabolism. This information will often help in the management of a patient with exercise intolerance or suspected heart or lung disease. Occasionally it is possible to demonstrate the absence of malfunction where symptoms have made the patient fear, and the clinician suspect, serious disease, leading to reassurance and advice.

The quantitative information may be of no specific structural or etiological significance. For any pattern of exercise response said to be diagnostic of a particular condition, it is not hard to find another diagnosis with which it is also compatible. As with most physiological tests, their usefulness is less in the diagnosis of structural abnormality than in the description of disturbed physiology which results from it. Usually it should be possible to relate the responses obtained in an exercise test to the demands made on the patient in his everyday life. Can he meet these demands without ill effect? In which direction may therapy best be directed to help him meet the demand? Should he adjust his life to lessen the demand?

The Diagnostic Uses of Exercise Testing

Having emphasized that the proper concern of physiological tests is with functional changes, we recognize that the problems which lead a clinician to ask for an investigation are couched more often in structural or causal than in functional terms: "What is causing this patient's symptoms and how bad is it?" rather than "What is the matter, how is it affecting function, and how is the body responding to it?" Physiological findings may have structural implications that can be useful, either because the response is diagnostic, or, more commonly, because the response indicates a functional abnormality which can be used diagnostically with other clinical information.

Conditions in which an exercise test may be diagnostic include the following:

- myocardial ischemia
- peripheral vascular disease

- exercise-induced asthma
- unfitness
- vasoregulatory asthenia
- psychogenic dyspnea
- muscle phosphorylase deficiency

We will not detail the abnormalities found in these conditions but would make a few observations at this point. Unfitness is common in urban men and women and may make the quantitative assessment of other conditions difficult. Psychogenic dyspnea is common in organic disease and can compound the physician's and the patient's assessment of severity. An exercise test will often allow an assessment to be made of the relative importance of unfitness or psychogenic dyspnea in a mixed situation.

There has been a recent tendency to suggest that arteriographic changes should replace other diagnostic criteria of myocardial ischemia. However, the presence of narrowing or obstruction of major coronary arteries may not be a reliable indication of inadequate myocardial blood flow, which is more realistically detected during excerise, when the myocardial oxygen needs are increased. The same arguments apply to peripheral vascular disease.

Muscle phosphorylase deficiency (McArdle's syndrome) is characterized by a severe exercise intolerance associated with an inability to break down glycogen: the recent introduction of muscle biopsy as a clinical tool may lead to the recognition of other defects in muscle enzyme activity.

CONDITIONS WHICH AN EXERCISE TEST CAN DETECT OR EXCLUDE

By this we mean conditions which, if present, will certainly cause an abnormal exercise response but which do not cause a diagnostic pattern of abnormality. Hence, in this category there should be no false negatives, but a positive result may be nonspecific. Virtually all diseases affecting the airways, lungs, pulmonary circulation, heart, systemic circulation, and blood could come under this category, but for the sake of clinical practice, the following is a conservative list of conditions in which abnormalities in an exercise test are likely to be diagnostically helpful.

- chronic bronchitis
- pulmonary emphysema
- pulmonary infiltration, alveolitis, and fibrosis

- pulmonary thromboembolism and hypertension
- congenital cardiac abnormalities
- cardiac valvular obstruction or incompetence
- primary myocardial disease

We reemphasize the concept that proper application of exercise tests is not so much in the narrower sense of diagnosis of these conditions but in a wider sense of assessing them. When used in this manner their diagnostic value may be increased indirectly in two ways. First, the response to exercise may be at variance with the clinical impression and may indicate the need for other investigations; for example, a patient thought to have asthma, in whom exercise reveals a cardiac limitation due to thromboembolic pulmonary hypertension. Secondly, exercise may allow a diagnostic weighting in a patient with more than one disorder; for example, a patient with valvular heart disease and chronic bronchitis, in whom the ventilatory impairment exceeds the cardiac, leading to a change in therapeutic emphasis.

THE USE OF EXERCISE TESTING IN CLINICAL MANAGEMENT

Many techniques used in clinical assessment become more valuable when repeated on several occasions in any one patient to follow the natural history of a condition or the effect of therapy. This is particularly true of exercise testing, in which a change in overall performance or in the performance of a single mechanism carries greater weight than an absolute value at a single point in time. One obvious application is in the use of regular exercise in rehabilitation programs. The initial exercise test will allow accurate prescription of the activity, so as to be safe yet effective, and also direct attention to mechanisms requiring particular care. Repeated testing will provide objective evidence of improvement and identify the mechanisms which underlie any change. It also provides a valuable tool for the physician to use in motivating the patient to continue the activity and in changing the activity to keep it at an optimal level. Many types of activity programs are in their infancy: assessment of their value must include objective evidence of improved function before they can be applied on a wider scale.

These are the general principles upon which we have developed the exercise testing procedures described in this book and the types of information that may be gained from their use. It remains to outline the scope of the chapters that follow. Although we have not divided the book into two parts, Chapters 2 and 3 contain material for the reader who wishes to find information regarding clinical exercise physiology and the use of exercise testing in clinical practice; Chapters 4, 5, and 6 are for those who wish to establish an exercise testing laboratory. Chapter 2 contains a brief account of the metabolic, cardiovascular, and respiratory adaptations to exercise and the effects of disease. Chapter 3 outlines exercise testing methods and the rationale behind the method we have adopted, in which CO_2 transport in the body is used to explore various mechanisms during exercise. Chapter 4 deals with the theory underlying the measurement of mixed venous carbon dioxide by an indirect rebreathing technique, which obviates the need for sampling blood from the right heart. Chapter 5 is concerned with the equipment required in an exercise testing laboratory, and Chapter 6 covers the detailed conduct of exercise testing in patients. Chapter 7 outlines the use that may be made of computers in exercise testing. Chapter 8 addresses itself to the problem of defining normal values for exercise test results. This is followed in Chapters 9, 10, and 11 by an approach to the interpretation of exercise test results, and some examples are given to expand this discussion in Chapter 12. The appendix defines terms and symbols, outlines calculations, and presents normal standards.

References

Campbell, E. J. M.: Exercise tolerance. Sci. Basis Med. Ann. Rev. 8:129-144, 1967.

Chapter Two

PHYSIOLOGY OF EXERCISE

The purpose of this chapter is to set the scene for what follows by briefly reviewing the physiology of muscular exercise in health and disease. Before doing so, some definitions and units of measurements require explanation, and the types of exercise considered later need to be described.

FORCE, WORK, AND POWER

The definition of unit force is that acting on unit mass to produce unit acceleration. The unit of force is that acting on a mass of one kg to produce an acceleration of $1 \text{ m} \cdot \text{sec}^2$ and is called the Newton (N). An object falling freely increases its speed by $9.80 \text{ m} \cdot \text{sec}^2$, and because the only force acting is gravity, the acceleration is constant. The gravitational force acting on a stationary mass of one kg is 9.80 N; this force is known as the kilopond (Kp).

The definition of unit work is that done when unit force acts through unit distance. A unit of work is done when a force of 1 N acts through 1 meter and is called one Newton-meter or one joule. If a mass of 1 kg is moved through a vertical distance of 1 m against the force of gravity, the work performed is 9.80 joules; this is more widely known as a kilopond-meter (kpm).

Throughout this book we will be concerned with dynamic exercise performed by large muscle groups. The external expression of this action is power, which is work performed per unit of time. As the unit of work is the joule, the unit of power is the joule per second, or watt (w). Many physiologists use the kpm as the unit of work, in which case the unit of power is the kilopond-meter per minute (kpm/

11

min). This equals $9.80 \div 60$ watts or 0.1635 w (an easier conversion to remember is that 600 kpm/min is about 100 w). Because physiologists have not reached agreement regarding which of these two units to use, we will usually express power outputs in both units.

For some purposes it may be important to express activity as a thermal equivalent in Kcal/min (1 Kcal/min = 427 kpm/min or 72 w). As there is a close relationship between power output and oxygen intake, most variables are related more logically to oxygen intake than power output. "METS" are units easily understood by patients and physicians in relation to everyday activity and the amount of exercise performed in "therapeutic" exercise programs; an MET is a multiple of the resting oxygen intake (3.5 ml O_2/kg/min).

Although the adoption of the S.I. system of notation has been well argued recently (Piiper, 1973), we have not used it in the text, but a table given in the Appendix allows the reader to convert measurements and symbols if required.

MUSCLE CONTRACTION AND ENERGY LIBERATION

In exercising man, work is done by shortening muscle. This is brought about in the myofibril by the sliding of thin actin filaments in between the thicker myosin filaments; the sliding is caused by the formation of cross-bridges, which produce the mechanical force (Needham, 1971; Murray and Weber, 1974). The formation of these bridges requires chemical energy, which is provided by the splitting of adenosine triphosphate (ATP).

Energy is dissipated as heat in isometric exercise even though no external work is performed. In the case of body movement, the application of forces through levers and the action of various frictional resistances lead to a complex relationship between the work performed by muscle and the external work produced. The efficiency of an engine is measured by the external work performed for a given internal energy dissipation, and similar measurements may be made in the case of the exercising human. Usually the energy equivalent of oxygen consumption is related to the power output to obtain the efficiency of muscular work, a value of 16 to 24 per cent being obtained (Wilkie, 1960).

Muscle contraction is dependent on a supply of ATP, which is present in low concentration in muscle (24μM/g dry muscle) and has to be resynthesized from ADP by a variety of mechanisms in order for contraction to continue.

1. *Phosphoryl creatine* exists in muscle at a higher concentration than ATP ($75\mu M/g$ dry weight) and provides a rapidly available source of high energy phosphate.

$$PC + ADP \longrightarrow C + ATP$$

   The equilibrium of this reaction favors the formation of ATP (Lohmann, 1935); levels of ATP in muscle fall only after stores of PC have been severely depleted (Hultman et al, 1967). PC itself is resynthesized by oxidative phosphorylation.

2. *Oxidative Phosphorylation.* A series of linked reactions allows the energy obtained from the oxidation of various fuels, mainly glycogen and free fatty acids, to be coupled to the uptake of inorganic phosphate in the resynthesis of ATP and PC. The series of oxidations involves transfer of electrons to an electron acceptor, or oxidizing agent. The principal electron acceptor is nicotinamide adenine dinucleotide (NAD), which thereby is reduced to NADH.

   The hydrogen of NADH is removed through two pathways. In the presence of oxygen, electrons are transferred along the electron carrier chain to molecular O_2:

$$NADH + H^+ + 1/2\ O_2 \longrightarrow NAD^+ + H_2O$$

In the absence of O_2, H^+ is accepted by pyruvate, formed from glycolysis, and lactate is produced:

$$pyruvate + NADH + H^+ \rightleftarrows lactate + NAD^+$$

   Although these two processes, aerobic and anaerobic, are for convenience described separately, they are invariably in dynamic equilibrium, their relative contribution to NAD resynthesis depending on the availability of oxygen. In this way, muscles are spared complete dependence on the mechanisms that deliver O_2 from air. This is of particular importance at the onset of exercise and in any situation where O_2 delivery to muscle is compromised, for example at altitude or in cardiopulmonary disease, because the O_2 delivery mechanisms take time to adapt to the demand. However, anaerobic glycolysis is far less effective in regenerating ATP than aerobic oxidation of carbohydrate or fat.

   The major metabolic pathways used to regenerate ATP are summarized in Figure 2–1 (for a more detailed description see Lehninger, 1970).

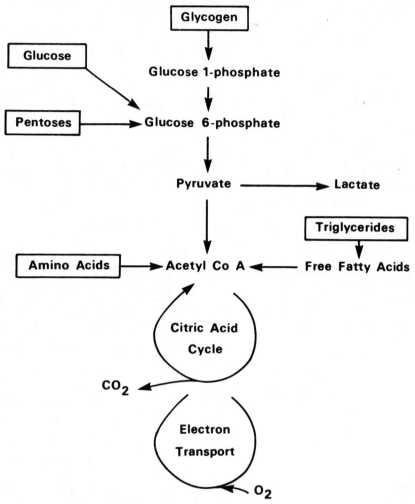

Figure 2–1   Main metabolic pathways used during exercise.

ENERGY YIELD FROM OXIDATION OF DIFFERENT FUELS

The relative yield of ATP molecules depends on whether aerobic or anaerobic processes are used and whether carbohydrate or fat is oxidized.

The equation describing the overall reaction for *anaerobic glycolysis* indicates that few ATP molecules are resynthesized from each glucosyl unit in glycogen:

(glycogen) glucose 6-P $+ 3 P_i + 3$ ADP $\longrightarrow$ 2 lactate $+ 3$ ATP $+ H_2O$

Starting from glucose, one less ATP molecule is made available owing to the usage of one ATP molecule in the formation of glucose 6-phosphate.

In contrast to anaerobic glycolysis, the *aerobic breakdown of glycogen* yields substantially more ATP:

(glycogen) glucose 6-P $+ 6 O_2 + 37 P_i + 37$ ADP $\longrightarrow$
$$6 CO_2 + 37 \text{ ATP} + H_2O$$

Free fatty acids are first esterified with coenzyme A (CoA) before crossing the mitochondrial membrane and being oxidized: for a representative free fatty acid (palmitic acid) the equation is as follows:

palmitoyl CoA $+ 23 O_2 + 131 P_i + 131$ ADP $\longrightarrow$
$$16 CO_2 + 131 \text{ ATP} + 146 H_2O$$

The oxidation of carbohydrates and fats is accompanied by a free-energy change, about 40 per cent of which is conserved by the formation of the energy-rich bonds of ATP and stored as potential energy until required for muscular contraction.

The Respiratory Quotient (R.Q.)

The R.Q. is the ratio of CO_2 produced to O_2 used during metabolism; from the preceding equations it can be seen that for the aerobic breakdown of glycogen the R.Q. is 1 (6/6) and of a free fatty acid it is 0.7 (16/23). Anaerobic glycolysis itself does not contribute to the R.Q. of muscle. However, lactic acid reacts with the bicarbonate of tissue fluids to produce carbonic acid, eventually leading to an increase in the total CO_2 evolution in the body. The ratio of CO_2 output to O_2 intake in the lungs is known as the respiratory exchange ratio (R). The distinction between the aerobic muscle R.Q. and the total body R will recur in several later chapters as well as below.

Factors Influencing the Type of Fuel
Used for Muscular Exercise

A variety of metabolic pathways are open to exercising muscle for the resynthesis of ATP. Although all may be used in any exercise, the emphasis in the pathways chosen will vary according to type of muscle fiber, severity and duration of exercise, and diet. The mechanisms involved have been reviewed exhaustively by Keul, Doll and Keppler (1972).

Variation in Metabolic Processes Among Types of Muscle

The source of energy for the resynthesis of ATP is not quantitatively the same in all muscles. In particular, the relative contribution of anaerobic and aerobic processes may vary considerably. The two extremes of this variation are seen in red muscle and white muscle (Gollnick et al, 1973). Red muscle fibers are slow contracting and involved in continuous or sustained activity; they are found in the flight muscles of birds and the antigravity muscles of mammals. They have a high content of myoglobin and mitochondrial enzymes, and a high capillary density; their metabolic demands are met mainly through aerobic processes. White muscles, on the other hand, are subject to less continuous activity, are fast contracting, have little myoglobin or respiratory enzymes, and glycolysis is the chief source of energy. Most skeletal muscles in humans are composed of both types of fiber, with a preponderance of red fibers in muscles that are in almost constant use such as the diaphragm and the postural muscles.

Usage of Anaerobic Processes

Circulatory and respiratory mechanisms have a limited capacity and also require time to increase sufficiently to meet oxygen demands, which are set by the muscles' power output. If the demand for oxygen outstrips the supply, for example at the onset of exercise or at a very high power output, the muscle makes use of local oxygen stores in myoglobin, stores of phosphoryl creatine, and anaerobic glycolysis. These local energy resources can support muscular activity for a short time only, after which muscle exhaustion will occur due to the failure of ATP resynthesis. At power outputs below exhaustive values, oxygen delivery eventually increases sufficiently to meet the demand, and local resources are replenished.

Anaerobic glycolysis leads to lactate production. It seems likely that even in healthy subjects some lactate is produced when muscle becomes active or increases its activity, but lactate in muscle does not increase significantly until an oxygen intake of about 50 per cent of the maximum is exceeded (Karlsson, 1971). Lactate does not diffuse

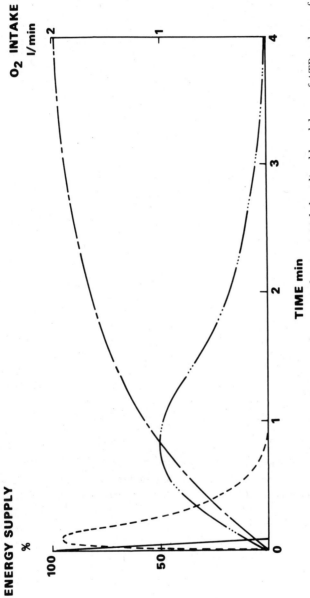

Figure 2-2 Sources of energy at the onset of exercise, showing initial short-lived breakdown of ATP and use of stored oxygen (—), breakdown of phosphoryl creatine (—·—), anaerobic glycolysis (— ·· —), and aerobic glycolysis (— – —).

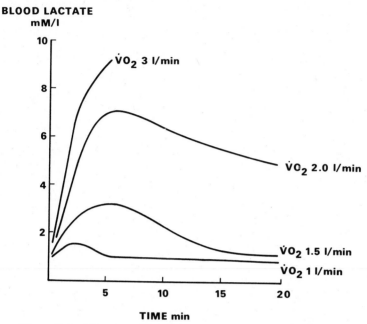

BLOOD LACTATE
  mM/l

$\dot{V}O_2$ 3 l/min

$\dot{V}O_2$ 2.0 l/min

$\dot{V}O_2$ 1.5 l/min

$\dot{V}O_2$ 1 l/min

TIME min

Figure 2-3 Changes in blood lactate found in one subject exercising at various power outputs.

from muscle rapidly, and a concentration gradient between tissue and blood may be present during a period of active lactate production, with the muscle lactate concentration being as high as 1.5 times that in blood. At a low power output, lactate in both muscle and blood increases transiently and then falls to resting levels (Figs. 2-2 and 2-3) owing to reduced production of lactate and its metabolism in inactive muscle, liver, and heart.

At the onset of exercise at a constant power output, there is a delay before a constant O_2 intake is achieved. This "oxygen deficit" is related to the increase in muscle lactate concentration and the fall in PC concentration (Karlsson, 1971). Similarly, at the end of exercise there is a delay before O_2 intake falls to resting levels: this increase in O_2 intake, the "oxygen debt," is presumably due to the replenishment of tissue O_2 stores, the aerobic metabolism of lactate, and resynthesis of muscle energy stores.

Unfortunately, the quantitative relationships between energy production, the biochemical processes, and the oxygen utilized are so complex and variable that the measurement of oxygen deficit and oxygen debt do not yield worthwhile information in clinical exercise testing. Changes in blood lactate, however, may be used as an indication of the inability of the oxygen delivery mechanisms to meet the demands of energy metabolism. In patients this may be due to impaired cardiovascular responses such as low cardiac output and slow adaptation at the onset of exercise, or to poor tissue perfusion in peripheral vascular disease. Less commonly, severe reduction in blood O_2 content due to pulmonary dysfunction, abnormal blood O_2 carriage, or an abnormality at the mitochondrial level, may lead to excessive use of anaerobic metabolic pathways.

It has long been held that high muscle lactate concentrations are directly related to exhaustion, but several observations suggest that this is not the only mechanism. In prolonged exercise terminated by maximal effort, for example in a long-distance race, lactate is not high (Åstrand et al, 1963). Local levels of lactate are not high in isolated muscle stimulated through its nerve to exhaustion. The highest levels of blood lactate (20 to 30 mM/L) are found with repeated spells of "supramaximal" exercise leading to exhaustion in less than 1 minute, alternating with rest periods of 4 to 5 minutes, during which PC and ATP are resynthesized before a significant quantity of lactate has been metabolized (Hermansen and Osnes, 1972). Although there may be several mechansims leading to muscle exhaustion, in exercise of short duration lactate accumulation is associated with a sensation of fatigue.

USAGE OF AEROBIC METABOLIC PATHWAYS

Information regarding the relative use of different fuels in aerobic exercise has come from a variety of experimental procedures, including measurement of the respiratory quotient (R.Q.); measurement of blood concentrations of metabolites; by use of radioactive tracer techniques; and, more recently, from microanalytical techniques applied to small samples of muscle obtained by needle biopsy.

The equations on page 15 show that the ratio of CO_2 production to O_2 utilization (R.Q.) is 1 in the case of glycogen and 0.7 in the case of a free fatty acid. Using this difference in R.Q., information has been obtained regarding the proportion of fats and carbohydrates used in muscular work, either in the body as a whole from measurements of O_2 and CO_2 in expired gas (Christensen and Hansen, 1939), or in an exercising limb from measurements of O_2 and CO_2 in arterial and venous blood (Andres et al, 1956). For the calculation of R.Q. to be valid, all the metabolic requirements must be met from aerobic metabolism, with no lactic acid being formed to generate CO_2, and stores of CO_2 and O_2 have to be in a steady state. These conditions are seldom fulfilled in patients, or in heavy exercise in healthy subjects, so that this indirect indication of fat and carbohydrate usage has a limited application.

At low work rates the R.Q. is usually about 0.85, indicating an equal usage of carbohydrate and fats. During exercise of short duration and increasing power output the R.Q. increases. A low R.Q. is found in work of long duration, particularly in the fasting state, when free fatty acids are used mainly. A meal causes an increase in R.Q. because of a reduced availability of free fatty acids, which is due to the inhibition of lipolysis in adipose tissue (Havel et al, 1963; Jones and Haddon, 1973).

The major carbohydrate fuel is glycogen stored in muscle. It has been shown that endurance in heavy exercise is closely related to muscle glycogen concentration. Muscle biopsies (Bergström et al, 1967) have shown also that glycogen levels fall sharply in heavy exercise due to anaerobic glycolysis; at lower work rates the fall is more gradual. This is due partly to the higher efficiency of aerobic glycolysis in regenerating ATP and partly to the higher use of free fatty acids. Although the turnover rate of glucose is increased during exercise, muscle uptake of glucose is small until exhausting levels of exercise are reached. Thus only about 10 per cent of the metabolic needs are supplied by glucose, unless blood glucose levels are high, for example following a high-carbohydrate meal. Following exercise, muscle glycogen is replenished, and if glycogen stores have been severely depleted, muscle glycogen increases during the next three days to above the pre-exercise level (Hultman, 1967).

The major source of fat for fuel in muscular exercise is adipose tissue; free fatty acids are liberated by the hydrolysis of triglycerides and transported, loosely bound, to plasma albumin. Uptake by muscle depends upon the muscle blood flow and the blood level of free fatty acids. The mobilization of free fatty acids takes time, blood levels of free fatty acids falling during the first 5 to 10 minutes of exercise, owing to the rapid uptake by muscle, and then steadily increasing due to mobilization. When exercise ceases, blood levels increase sharply as a result of the reduction in muscle uptake. Mobilization of free fatty acids is under complex hormonal control; catecholamines increase lipase activity in adipose tissue, and insulin exerts a powerful effect on free fatty acid mobilization that almost ceases following a meal or a glucose infusion (Havel, 1965).

Hydrolysis of triglycerides in adipose tissue yields free glycerol, which cannot be reused, and leads to an increase in blood glycerol level; metabolism of glycerol occurs mainly in the liver. The part played by fatty acids obtained from triglycerides stored in the muscle cell is uncertain. Although this source has been thought to contribute little to muscle metabolism, recent studies employing a biopsy technique suggest that it may be used when the supply of free fatty acids from blood is reduced (Carlson et al, 1971).

Although amino acids and ketoacids can be used by exercising muscle, their contribution is quantitatively small (Felig and Wahren, 1971).

From this brief review it can be appreciated that the factors influencing the choice of fuels are complex and difficult to define precisely in all situations. Power output, duration of exercise, and diet are the most important factors. However, the ability of a muscle to use several fuels gives it a flexibility in maintaining ATP supply in a wide variety of situations. In heavy exercise, muscle glycogen is mainly used, anaerobic glycolysis being particularly important at the onset; thereafter aerobic glycolysis is dominant. In moderate exercise of longer duration half the needs are met by oxidation of carbohydrates (about 40 per cent from glycogen and 10 per cent from glucose) and half by free fatty acids (about 40 per cent from adipose tissue stores and 10 per cent from muscle fat) (Havel et al, 1967; Carlson et al, 1971). In exercise of several hours' duration, free fatty acids are used to an increasing extent (Young et al, 1967).

Ill health may influence the metabolic adaptations to exercise in a number of ways. Inactivity may lead to reduced levels of mitochondrial enzymes and energy stores, and interference with oxygen delivery leads to a greater use of anaerobic mechanisms. In addition, a few rare conditions are recognized in which absence of specific intramuscular enzymes affects the ability to perform exercise. The best studied example is that of McArdle's syndrome, in which muscle phosphorylase is absent. Because this enzyme catalyzes the breakdown of glycogen to glucose-1-phosphate, glycogen cannot be used for energy metabolism. For this reason, these patients are dependent upon the supply of free fatty acids and glucose to muscle. The characteristic features are an inability to do heavy work, the absence of lactate in blood from working muscle, and the presence of a "second wind" phenomenon in which a gradual "warm-up" allows a work rate to be performed which is higher than that without warming up. This warm-up presumably leads to an increase in blood flow and delivery of free fatty acids and glucose (Pernow et al, 1967). The severe limitation in exercise tolerance which these patients experience emphasizes the importance of normal glycogen metabolism in exercise.

PULMONARY ADAPTATIONS TO EXERCISE

Ventilation, pulmonary gas transfer, cardiac output, and peripheral blood flow all increase in response to the metabolic demands of

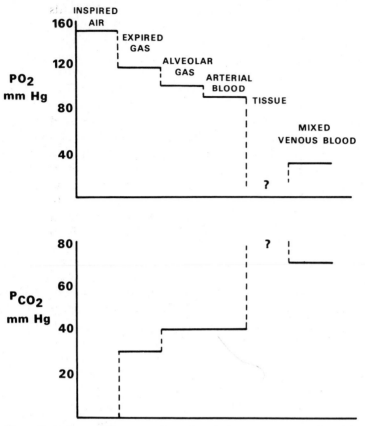

Figure 2-4 P_{O_2} and P_{CO_2} at various sites during exercise at an O_2 intake of 2 L/min.

working muscles. In disease, structural changes may interfere with these adaptations, causing reduced exercise tolerance, but various mechanisms help to compensate, tending to maintain O_2 supply and CO_2 excretion. Often a patient's symptoms are related more to the compensatory mechanisms than to the initiating abnormality.

The transfer of oxygen from air to muscle cell and of CO_2 in the reverse direction can be considered as a series of cascades in which various mechanisms influence the differences in CO_2 and O_2 pressures in various sites (Fig. 2–4).

Pulmonary Ventilation, Blood Flow, and Gas Exchange

The mathematical relationships involved in the series of mechanisms illustrated in Figure 2–4 will be examined before the changes which occur in exercise are described. Although each of these mechanisms may be considered in relation to both O_2 and CO_2, either may be chosen according to convention, for physiological reasons, or for reasons related to measurement.

Pulmonary ventilation ($\dot{V}_E$) and its subdivisions — alveolar ventilation ($\dot{V}_A$) and "dead space" ventilation ($\dot{V}_D$) — are expressed in terms of CO_2. The relationship between ventilation and CO_2 output is expressed in terms of the mixed expired CO_2 concentration ($F_E CO_2$) —

$$F_E CO_2 = \frac{\dot{V}_{CO_2}}{\dot{V}_E}$$

Or, where expired CO_2 is expressed as a partial pressure:

$$P_E CO_2 = \frac{\dot{V}_{CO_2} \times K}{\dot{V}_E} \qquad \textbf{Equation 1}$$

In this equation K converts fractional concentration to partial pressure and corrects $\dot{V}_E$ to conditions at body temperature (BTPS): K is 0.863 when $\dot{V}_{CO_2}$ is expressed in ml/min STPD and $\dot{V}_E$ in L/min BTPS, at a barometric pressure of 760 mm Hg and temperature 37°C.

Similarly, alveolar ventilation for a given CO_2 output is defined by the alveolar P_{CO_2},

$$F_A CO_2 = \frac{\dot{V}_{CO_2}}{\dot{V}_A}$$

or

$$P_A CO_2 = \frac{\dot{V}_{CO_2} \times 0.863}{\dot{V}_A} \qquad \textbf{Equation 2}$$

Following the mathematical analysis of alveolar gas composition by Riley and Cournand (1949), arterial P_{CO_2} has been used as the closest "effective" estimate of the "ideal" alveolar P_{CO_2}, representative of lung regions taking part in gas exchange.

$$P_a CO_2 = \frac{\dot{V}_{CO_2} \times 0.863}{\dot{V}_A} \qquad \textbf{Equation 3}$$

Although this concept may be challenged on theoretical grounds because abnormalities in the distribution of ventilation-perfusion ratios will lead to a difference between the P_{CO_2} of mixed alveolar gas and arterial blood, the effect is small and does not lead to important errors in clinical exercise testing (Farhi, 1966). If necessary a correction may be applied using a second approximation procedure (Riley and Cournand, 1951), an example of which is given on p. 172.

The remainder of the ventilation is considered to be wasted, as if it were distributed to areas receiving inspired air but no blood. The total or "physiological" dead space has two components – the airway dead space and the alveolar dead space due to the high ventilation: perfusion ratio of lung regions. Physiological dead space is expressed as the dead space:tidal volume (V_D/V_T) ratio, calculated by an equation first used by Christian Bohr (1889):

$$\frac{V_D}{V_T} = \frac{P_aCO_2 - P_ECO_2}{P_aCO_2 - P_ICO_2}$$ **Equation 4**

In this equation, the inspired CO_2 (P_ICO_2) is assumed to be so small (0.4 mm Hg) that it can be ignored.

The total blood flow ($\dot{Q}_t$) is defined by Fick's principle:

$$\dot{Q}_t = \frac{\dot{V}O_2}{C_aO_2 - C_{\bar{v}}O_2}$$ **Equation 5**

where C_aO_2 and $C_{\bar{v}}O_2$ are the concentration of O_2 in arterial and mixed venous blood respectively. In the same way that ventilation was subdivided into alveolar and dead space portions, the total blood flow may be subdivided into the pulmonary capillary blood flow, taking part in gas exchange, and a portion which is "wasted" with regard to gas exchange, either because it passes from the right to left heart through an anatomical pathway or because it flows through areas in which the ventilation:perfusion ratio is low or alveolar–capillary O_2 transfer impaired. This portion is expressed as the venous admixture ratio,

$$\frac{\dot{Q}_{va}}{\dot{Q}_t} = \frac{C_cO_2 - C_aO_2}{C_cO_2 - C_{\bar{v}}O_2}$$ **Equation 6**

The similarity to the V_D/V_T ratio should be noted: Equation 6 calculates the extent to which the pulmonary end-capillary O_2 (C_cO_2) is altered by admixture of venous blood ($C_{\bar{v}}O_2$) to lead to the O_2 content in mixed arterial blood.

The ideal alveolar PO_2 determines the ideal end-capillary O_2 content, and the arterial O_2 content determines the arterial PO_2. For this reason the alveolar-arterial PO_2 difference is used as a reflection of venous admixture; arterial PO_2 is measured and alveolar PO_2 calculated using the alveolar air equation, a simplified form of which is as follows:

$$P_AO_2 = P_IO_2 - \frac{P_aCO_2}{R}$$ **Equation 7**

However, an increase in the A-a P_{O_2} difference should be interpreted with caution in exercise as it may not indicate an increased venous admixture. Changes in alveolar ventilation (and thus in P_aCO_2) will influence P_AO_2 (Equation 7) and thus $C_{\acute{c}}O_2$ (Equation 6); changes in cardiac output will influence $C_{\bar{v}}O_2$ (Equation 5) and thus will alter C_aO_2 for a given value of $\dot{Q}_{va}/\dot{Q}_t$ (Equation 6). A wide A-a P_{O_2} difference may thus be the result of alveolar hyperventilation and a low cardiac output rather than of a high $\dot{Q}_{va}/\dot{Q}_t$ ratio and therefore does not necessarily imply an abnormal dispersion of ventilation: perfusion ratios or impaired alveolar–capillary oxygen transfer.

The two ratios, V_D/V_T and $\dot{Q}_{va}/\dot{Q}_t$, are used as indices of pulmonary gas exchange efficiency rather than as quantitative measurements of the dead space volume or amount of right-to-left shunting of blood in the lungs. It should be borne in mind that this use of the two ratios handles the complex relationships involved in pulmonary gas exchange in a simplistic way, in which the lung behaves as a three-compartment model. Although the approach may be criticized for this reason, and more complex models may be developed in the future, this method allows the gas exchange abnormality in patients to be usefully quantified and has stood the test of utility for 28 years (Farhi, 1966).

The preceding equations will recur in graphical form below in considering the changes that occur in exercise.

Ventilation, Tidal Volume, and the Frequency of Breathing

Ventilation increases in a linear relationship to O_2 intake and CO_2 output up to power outputs of 50 to 60 per cent of the maximal VO_2 above this, ventilation is more closely related to CO_2 output, which increases to a greater extent than O_2 intake. The P_{CO_2} of mixed expired gas (P_ECO_2) increases to a maximum at about 75 per cent of the maximal power output, above which P_ECO_2 falls (Fig. 2–5). The linear portion of the ventilatory response is expressed by the following equation, obtained from studies in healthy subjects (Jones 1964):

$$\dot{V}_E = 4.54 + .0221\ \dot{V}_{CO_2}\ (\text{S.D. } 2.50)$$

where $\dot{V}_E$ is expressed in l/min BTPS and $\dot{V}_{CO_2}$ in ml/min STPD. Within this relationship there is variation among subjects, which is related to differences in the ventilatory response to a CO_2 stimulus (Rebuck et al, 1973). As expressed in Equations 1 to 3 (p. 23),

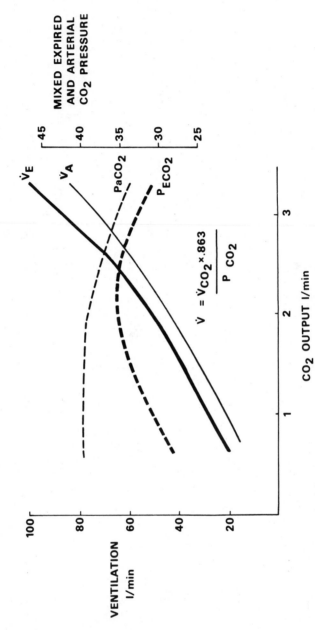

$$\dot{V} = \frac{\dot{V}_{CO_2} \times .863}{P\ CO_2}$$

Figure 2–5   The ventilatory response to exercise. The thick solid line shows mean total ventilation ($\dot{V}_E$) and thin line alveolar ventilation ($\dot{V}_A$). Dotted lines show mean values for P_aCO_2 and P_ECO_2.

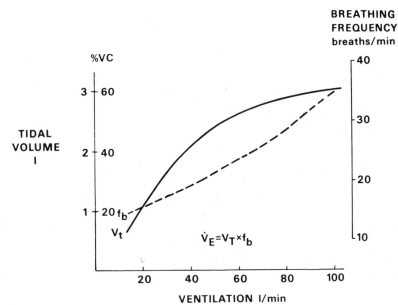

Figure 2–6 Tidal volume and breathing frequency in normal males. The graph may be applied to all subjects by expressing V_T as % VC and ventilation as % maximum ventilation instead of L/min.

P_ECO_2 and P_aCO_2 express the response of total (V_E) and alveolar ventilation (V_A) to metabolic CO_2 production. At submaximal power outputs P_aCO_2 remains relatively constant, indicating that $\dot{V}_A$ increases in proportion to $\dot{V}CO_2$. However, P_ECO_2 shows a rise towards P_aCO_2, indicating that $\dot{V}_E$ approaches $\dot{V}_A$ during exercise, owing to a fall in dead space ventilation, as detailed below. P_ECO_2 falls in heavy exercise owing to an increase in $\dot{V}_A$, shown by the parallel fall in P_aCO_2.

It follows from the relationships expressed in Equations 1 to 4 that changes in ventilation should be considered in terms of changes in alveolar ventilation and the V_D/V_T ratio. A ventilation that is high for a given power output, if not due to an increase in $\dot{V}CO_2$, is an indication of an increase in either or both. On the other hand, a reduced total ventilation implies alveolar hypoventilation. It is also apparent that a normal ventilation may be accounted for by a low alveolar ventilation and increased V_D/V_T ratio.

In healthy subjects the increase in ventilation at low levels of work is due mainly to an increase in the tidal volume. The relationship between V_T and V_E is hyperbolic, V_T increasing to an asymptote at 60 to 70 per cent of the vital capacity (Fig. 2–6) (Rebuck et al, 1974). The shape of this curve appears to be determined by the hyperbolic relationship between volume and transpulmonary pressure and seems to optimize the mean force developed by respiratory muscles at any given level of ventilation. In healthy children, lung volumes are smaller than in adults, and the increase in ventilation is brought about more by an increase in the breathing frequency, values of up to 60 breaths/min being observed commonly.

In patients with a reduced lung volume the increase in ventilation during exercise is associated with high breathing frequencies and low tidal volumes, a finding which may be diagnostically useful. This breathing pattern is due mainly to mechanical factors (Rebuck et al, 1974). The low tidal volume may also compromise gas exchange in these patients, by increasing the V_D/V_T ratio.

Patients with chronic airway obstruction, on the other hand, breathe with low frequencies and with tidal volumes that may be surprisingly high when considered in relation to measurements of airway obstruction such as the one-second forced expired volume (FEV_1). Ventilatory capacity is limited by airflow in these patients, and the pattern of breathing adopted by them minimizes the work of breathing. When the demands of exercise require levels of ventilation that cannot be met with an economical pattern of breathing, tidal volume falls and the sensation of dyspnea increases.

In considering a ventilatory limit to exercise, the values obtained during exercise may be related to the maximal ventilation that can be sustained voluntarily. For many years the index used for this value has been the maximum breathing capacity (MBC) as measured over 15 seconds. This "sprint" value is larger than the ventilation that can be maintained voluntarily for 1 to 4 minutes, a period more applicable to exercise. The maximal ventilation sustained voluntarily for 4 minutes (4 min MVV) has been extensively studied by Freedman (1970), who showed that it could be predicted in healthy subjects from the FEV_1 using the following equation:

$$MVV = 129 + 25 \ (FEV_1 - 4.01) \ L/min$$

This relationship is approximated by $35 \times FEV_1$, which will also predict the MVV in patients with moderate ventilatory impairment. In most healthy subjects the ventilation in maximal exercise will reach values of around 70 per cent of the MVV. However, in patients with airway obstruction, ventilation during maximal exercise may equal the MVV, indicating that a ventilatory limit has been reached (Clark et al, 1969). Patients with severe airway obstruction (FEV_1 less than one liter) commonly achieve a maximal exercise ventilation which exceeds the $FEV_1 \times 35$ (Jones et al, 1971).

At a very high ventilation, the work of the respiratory muscles may increase to levels at which the sensation of dyspnea is intolerable.

Furthermore, at ventilations above 120 L/min in normal subjects, the increase in oxygen intake achieved by an increase in ventilation is offset almost entirely by the oxygen requirements of the respiratory muscles (Shephard, 1966). This may occur at a much lower ventilation in patients with abnormal lungs, in whom the work of breathing is greater.

Alveolar Ventilation

In health, arterial P_{CO_2} during exercise varies little from its resting values and seldom rises more than 1 to 2 mm Hg. Thus, by implication, at low and moderate levels of work, alveolar ventilation increases linearly with CO_2 output (Equation 2) (Fig. 2–5). The range of arterial P_{CO_2} during exercise is 35 to 45 mm Hg in healthy subjects. We will not consider all the factors thought to play a part in the control of breathing during exercise; in addition to neurogenic factors, changes in CO_2, O_2, and pH also stimulate breathing, and complex mathematical expressions have been derived to describe their effects quantitatively (Cunningham, 1963). Above 75 per cent of the maximum $\dot{V}O_2$, arterial P_{CO_2} shows a progressive fall, indicating that alveolar ventilation is increasing out of proportion to CO_2 output. Because the work rate at which this occurs is that at which a rise in blood lactate is seen, it is generally considered that the alveolar hyperventilation at high workloads is due primarily to the effect of a fall in arterial pH.

A low arterial P_{CO_2} is a common finding in patients with diffuse pulmonary infiltrative and fibrotic conditions, unless the ventilatory capacity is grossly impaired. The stimulus for alveolar hyperventilation is caused, at least in part, by a fall in arterial P_{O_2}. An impaired cardiovascular response to exercise is also associated with hyperventilation; this is due partly to lactic acidemia. In some cardiac diseases pulmonary hypertension appears to be responsible for hyperventilation. Severe hyperventilation associated with arterial P_{CO_2} of 20 to 25 mm Hg characteristically occurs during exercise in patients with obstructive pulmonary vascular disease (Jones and Goodwin, 1965). The observation of a reduction in ventilation and frequency following vagal blockade in such patients suggests that vagally mediated reflexes in the lungs or pulmonary circulation may be important (Guz et al, 1970).

Patients with severe and chronic airway obstruction often exhibit a rise in P_aCO_2 with exercise, sometimes amounting to 20 mm Hg or more (Jones, 1966). This is probably due to a combination of an increased effort to breathe and a reduced central responsiveness to

CO_2. The rise in P_{CO_2} generally is higher in patients with chronic obstructive bronchitis than in those with panlobular emphysema.

The V_D/V_T Ratio

The V_D/V_T ratio is normally 25 to 35 per cent at rest and falls to values between 5 and 20 per cent during exercise (Jones et al, 1966). The increased efficiency of ventilation brought about by this fall leads to a narrowing of the difference between P_aCO_2 and P_ECO_2 (Fig. 2–5). The fall in V_D/V_T is due to two competing effects. First, an increase in tidal volume tends to reduce the V_D/V_T ratio. Secondly, increases in end inspiratory volume and transpulmonary pressure tend to increase the anatomical dead space, but this effect is small (Fig. 2–7). Although in healthy subjects at rest in the upright position there is a small contribution to the V_D/V_T ratio from alveolar dead space, caused by the relative underperfusion of apical regions of the lung, this disappears during exercise, when lung perfusion becomes more even and apical areas become well perfused (West, 1963).

The V_D/V_T ratio may be increased in disease for several reasons. First, a small tidal volume increases the V_D/V_T ratio. Secondly, the presence of high ventilation:perfusion ratios in the lungs leads to "alveolar" dead space. The highest values for the V_D/V_T ratio (greater than 50 per cent) are seen in patients with diffuse pulmonary fibrotic conditions, in whom the tidal volume is very small and ventilation:

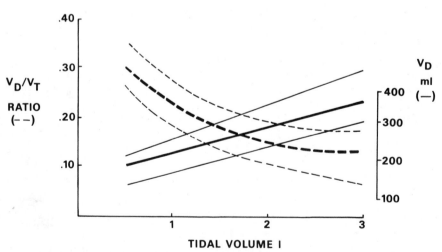

Figure 2–7   Physiological dead space (V_D) and the V_D/V_T ratio, mean values for males (thick lines) and range (thin lines).

perfusion relationships grossly abnormal. Widespread disease of the pulmonary vessels may lead to poor perfusion of large areas of lung, causing a marked increase in the V_D/V_T ratio. High V_D/V_T ratios are also observed in patients with severe chronic airway obstruction, but because of the alveolar underventilation, the total ventilation is often normal (Jones, 1964). Thus a normal value for the total ventilation should not be taken to indicate a normal pulmonary response to exercise without ensuring (through measurement of arterial or mixed venous Pco_2) that it is not due to a combination of these two abnormalities.

Venous Admixture

The A-a Po_2 difference is normally about 10 mm Hg at rest because of lung regions with a low ventilation:perfusion ratio. During exercise at low workloads it does not change, but at heavy workloads there is an increase to about 30 mm Hg (Fig. 2–8) (Jones et al, 1966). Because the mixed venous O_2 content falls during exercise, the finding of an unchanged A-a Po_2 difference during moderate work indicates an improvement in O_2 transfer in the lung (fall in $\dot{Q}_{va}/\dot{Q}_t$ ratio). This improvement is due to a more even distribution of ventilation: perfusion ratios in the lung (West, 1963; Hesser and Matell, 1965). An increase in A-a Po_2 during heavy work is the result of a rise in P_AO_2 owing to alveolar overventilation, and of a low venous O_2 content; a variable but small contribution due to incomplete alveolar–capillary O_2 equilibration may also be present (McHardy, 1972).

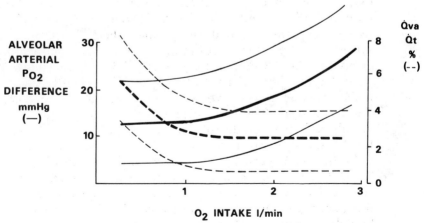

Figure 2–8 The alveolar-arterial Po_2 difference and venous admixture ($\dot{Q}_{va}/\dot{Q}_t$). Mean values for males (thick lines) ±2 SD (thin lines).

Impaired pulmonary O_2 transfer leads to an increase in the A-a PO_2 difference during exercise, which may be an early indication of abnormality, present before resting pulmonary function measurements are abnormal. Such an increase has been found in asymptomatic cigarette smokers, presumably due to disease of small airways (Levine et al, 1970), and also in the early stages of diffuse alveolitis. Reduced ventilation of well-perfused areas in the lung is the main cause of an increased A-a PO_2 difference at rest in many patients. During exercise the ventilation of these areas will often increase owing to an increase in tidal volume, resulting in a fall both in the A-a PO_2 difference and the $\dot{Q}_{va}/\dot{Q}_t$ ratio. This occurs in patients with chronic airway obstruction due to chronic bronchitis (Jones, 1966). Thus a wide A-a PO_2 difference at rest, although indicative of abnormal function, cannot be taken to signify an irreversible structural limitation to pulmonary O_2 uptake. However, in emphysema and pulmonary fibrosis, gas exchange does not improve with exercise; very wide A-a PO_2 differences are usually found in these conditions associated with falls in arterial PO_2.

Patients with a low cardiac output may show an increase in the A-a PO_2 difference during exercise even when pulmonary gas exchange processes are normal, because of the low mixed venous O_2 content: $\dot{Q}_{va}/\dot{Q}_t$ is normal unless pulmonary changes are present.

OXYGEN TRANSPORT IN BLOOD

The amount of oxygen carried by blood is dependent on the hemoglobin (Hb) concentration, the arterial PO_2, and the affinity of Hb for oxygen. The shape of the oxygen dissociation curve allows a high proportion of oxygen unloading for the change in oxygen tension in the tissue capillaries. Several factors may affect this during exercise, including temperature, arterial pH, arterial PCO_2, and concentration of erythrocyte 2,3 diphosphoglycerate (2,3 DPG). Of these, the first three are rapid and equal to the Bohr effect. The last has received much attention in recent years but seems unlikely to be of importance during exercise. The level of 2,3 DPG formed in the red cells by glycolysis has a unique role in the regulation of oxygen transport: it shifts the O_2 dissociation curve to the right and thus allows greater unloading of oxygen in the tissues. Although increased values of 2,3 DPG have been found in conditions associated with hypoxemia, cardiac disease, and anemia (Lenfant et al, 1969; Shapell et al, 1970), the quantitative importance of this mechanism in the maintenance of O_2 delivery during exercise has yet to be established.

In patients with anemia, an increase in cardiac output maintains O_2 delivery, and it is only when anemia is severe (Hb below 8 g/100 ml), or a cardiac impairment coexists, that effort symptoms become prominent. Studies of blood removal and reinfusion in athletes appear to show that maximal O_2 uptake can be directly related to the total available Hb (Ekblom et al, 1972). Further evidence for the importance of the functionally available mass of Hb has been provided by studies in which the O_2 capacity of Hb was reduced by carbon monoxide administration (Ekblom and Huot, 1972). However, these studies are in conflict with others which have shown that changes in total body Hb have little or no effect on maximal O_2 intake; the evidence has been reviewed recently by Rowell (1974).

CARDIOVASCULAR ADAPTATIONS TO EXERCISE

Cardiac Output

In health, cardiac output during exercise is linearly related to oxygen uptake (Fig. 2–9) (Eq. 5). Although at rest cardiac output is related to body size, this is probably dependent on the relationship between oxygen intake and size; during exercise the change in cardiac

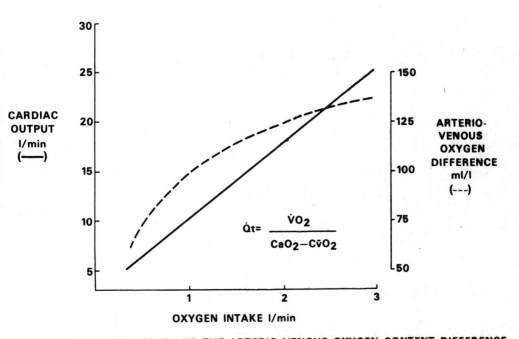

$$\dot{Q}t = \frac{\dot{V}O_2}{CaO_2 - C\bar{v}O_2}$$

CARDIAC OUTPUT AND THE ARTERIO VENOUS OXYGEN CONTENT DIFFERENCE

Figure 2–9 Cardiac output and the arteriovenous O_2 difference: mean values for males.

output for a given change in O₂ uptake is little affected by such factors as sex, age, and size. Pooled results from a large number of studies (Wade and Bishop, 1962) in a variety of subjects exercising in the erect posture have shown that the relationship may be expressed by the equation

$$\dot{Q}_t = 4 + .006\ \dot{V}O_2\ (\pm\ SD\ 2)\ L/min$$

where $\dot{V}O_2$ is expressed in ml/min. Values 2 L/min above this are found in the supine position (Bevegård et al, 1960, 1963). The increase in cardiac output is brought about mainly by an increase in cardiac frequency, which rises linearly with $\dot{V}O_2$ (Fig. 2–10). Maximal frequency is influenced primarily by age. This is the main reason for the decline in maximal oxygen uptake that occurs with advancing age; at an age of 20 years maximum frequency is 170 to 210, but it declines to 150 to 180 at the age of 60. The maximum cardiac frequency (obtained from many published studies reviewed by Lange-Anderson et al., 1971) is expressed by the following equation (see Fig. 2–11):

$$Max\ f_c = 210 - 0.65 \times age\ (yrs)$$

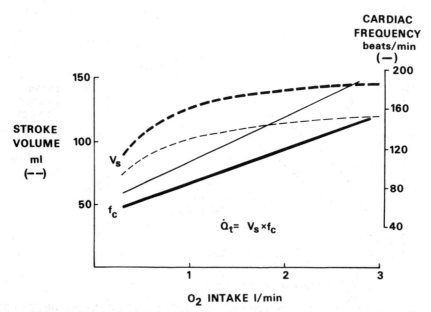

Figure 2-10 Stroke volume and cardiac frequency, comparing results obtained in an athlete (thick lines) and an untrained male (thin lines).

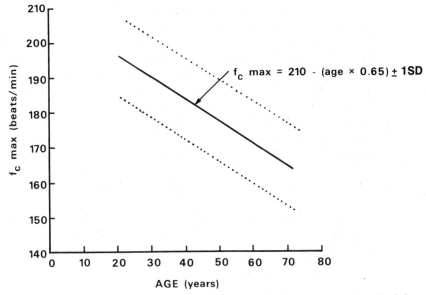

f_c max = 210 - (age × 0.65) ± **1SD**

Figure 2-11   Maximum cardiac frequency in normal adults.

Stroke Volume

Cardiac stroke volume increases to above resting values at low levels of work, but there is little or no further increase once cardiac frequency has risen to 120 beats/min (Fig. 2–10). The increase in stroke volume is brought about partly by an increased ventricular filling due to increased venous return and partly by enhanced contractility of the myocardium. Greater ventricular emptying leads to a fall in the end diastolic volume.

Stroke volume in health is mainly dependent on heart size, which therefore is an important factor influencing maximal cardiac output. This explains the accuracy with which heart size, determined radiographically, can be used to predict maximum O_2 uptake (Sjöstrand, 1960) and probably also accounts for the dependence of the heart rate–oxygen uptake relationship on body size. Stroke volumes are larger in men than women and in athletes than in untrained subjects (Fig. 2–10) (Bevegård et al, 1963), both findings being explained to a great extent, but not entirely, by differences in heart size.

Patients with mild degrees of valvular heart disease may maintain a normal stroke volume but usually at the expense of an increase in ventricular volume and in end diastolic pressure. These changes may contribute to the maintenance of a normal relationship between cardiac output and oxygen intake, but in more severe degrees of valvular dysfunction, stroke volume falls. At this stage an increased heart rate response to a given O_2 intake is found; the increase in cardiac frequency is seldom sufficient to maintain a normal cardiac output in this situation, and the maximum cardiac output is low (Werkö, 1964). If the cardiac output response to increasing O_2 intake is low, tissue O_2 uptake may be maintained by an increase in extraction of oxygen from blood, resulting in a low O_2 content in venous blood. Again, this adaptation is seldom complete; anaerobic metabolism occurs, leading to higher than normal levels for blood lactate concentration (Sjöstrand, 1960). A further problem facing such patients is the competition between working muscles and essential organs such as the kidney, or, particularly if there is a thermal stress, the skin, which normally operate at a high flow in relation to their metabolic rate. Thus the highest a-v O_2 differences are not found in such patients (see below). Patients with heart disease also may show a slow rate of adaptation of cardiac output to exercise, leading to an accentuation of the normal accumulation of lactic acid at the onset of exercise.

In patients with ischemic heart disease, stroke volume is often maintained, but left ventricular end-diastolic pressure usually increases (Parker, 1967). The onset of angina pectoris during exercise appears to be related to the myocardial oxygen requirements ($M\dot{V}o_2$). These are determined by the length:tension relationships of ventricular muscle and the heart rate (Sonnenblick et al, 1965) and are reflected clinically by measurements of the double product (systolic BP × heart rate) or triple product (systolic BP × heart rate × systolic ejection time). Although there is wide variation among patients in the relationship between these products and ST segment depression, they are helpful in assessing $M\dot{V}o_2$ in a given patient. For example, Redwood et al (1972) have shown that training may lead to an increase in the power output at which angina occurs, through reduction in BP and cardiac frequency, without any change in the triple product at which angina occurs. The same authors were also able to show that the triple product at angina is increased by treatment with coronary vasodilators and coronary bypass surgery. It is not uncommon in patients with ischemic heart disease to find that heart rate is low for a given power output or O_2 intake; the heart rate at maximal work is also low but is accompanied by a high blood lactate, suggesting that the cardiac output has reached limiting values. This response suggests that ischemia has led to a disturbance of the chronotropic properties of the myocardium, and a similar response is seen in patients being treated with a beta blocking drug such as propranolol. Such patients are usually found to have severe coronary atherosclerosis affecting the right and circumflex coronary arteries. This finding means that a target heart rate based on the maximal rate found in healthy subjects may be unrealistically high for many patients with ischemic heart disease. The electrocardiographic changes found in such patients is discussed in a later chapter (p. 107).

Poor exercise performance in patients with heart disease may be difficult to distinguish from the effects of inactivity. It has been shown that healthy subjects spending three weeks in bed have a reduced stroke volume, leading to a severe reduction in exercise performance, which takes several weeks to recover (Saltin et al, 1968).

Cardiac Rhythm

An abnormality of cardiac rhythm may limit exercise by changing ventricular filling time, and thus stroke volume. Atrial fibrillation is usually associated with a very limited stroke volume, which may be increased by digitalis. Atrioventricular dissociation, for example in congenital or acquired heart block, may lead to very low and relatively fixed heart rates. In spite of this, exercise performance may be surprisingly well maintained owing to high stroke volumes and increased peripheral O_2 extraction (Segal et al, 1964; Edhag and Zetterquist, 1968). Ectopic beats present at rest may become less frequent during exercise. However, exercise may also provoke abnormalities of cardiac rhythm or conduction. In a population survey of nearly 800 men, Vedin and co-workers (1972) found rhythm disturbances in 11.7 per cent of subjects. The most common arrhythmia provoked by exercise was ventricular premature beats; their presence correlated with electrocardiographic changes of myocardial ischemia and, when frequent, were related to an increased incidence of sudden death. Frequent ventricular premature beats may lead to ventricular tachycardia and fibrillation during exercise, which generally respond rapidly to counter-shock therapy. Other disturbances are less common (Gooch, 1972): paroxysmal atrial tachycardia and fibrillation are rarely encountered and usually revert following cessation of exercise. Bundle branch block appears to be rate-related, occurring only above a certain cardiac frequency and settling when frequency drops to below this critical value.

Arteriovenous Oxygen Difference

The arteriovenous oxygen difference is dependent on the completeness of oxygen extraction from blood by muscle. This in turn is influenced by the metabolic rate; regional distribution of peripheral flow; local muscle capillary density and perfusion; changes in the position of the O_2 dissociation curve; and probably the activity of muscle respiratory enzymes. Because maximal cardiac output is dependent on relatively fixed mechanisms governing stroke volume and heart rate, these factors assume important roles in determining maximum O_2 intake in both health and disease. When they are poorly developed, work performance may be impaired.

In health, the a-v O_2 content difference widens with increasing O_2 uptake from a resting level of around 50 ml/L to about 130 to 150 ml/L, the O_2 saturation of venous blood approaching 25–35 per cent in maximal work (Fig. 2–9). In trained athletes venous oxygen saturation may fall to 10–20 per cent (Pernow, Wahren and Zetterquist, 1965). These figures indicate a high utilization of transported oxygen in muscle, which is brought about by redistribution of blood to working tissue; up to 80 per cent of the increase in cardiac output during exercise is directed to muscle. Blood flow to brain and kidneys changes little during exercise, but flow to the liver and splanchnic region falls (Fig. 2–12) (Rowell et al, 1965). Skin perfusion is also reduced unless work is performed in high environmental temperatures, when it may amount to up to a quarter of the total cardiac output (Shephard, 1969).

In patients with a cardiac limitation to exercise, more complete extraction of oxygen from blood perfusing muscle assumes an important role in the maintenance of oxygen delivery. Although the arteriovenous O_2 difference at a given O_2 intake is often increased, it seldom reaches the highest levels seen in athletes at maximum effort, probably because of the competition from essential organs having a high blood flow relative to their metabolic rate. Although their absolute blood flow may be small, it makes up a greater proportion of the total cardiac output. However, it would be naive to consider the arteriovenous O_2 difference or the venous O_2 content as being influenced by the ratio of cardiac output to metabolic rate only; distribution of blood flow between organs and tissues and the balance between mean blood pressure and peripheral vascular resistance are factors whose importance is difficult to quantify (Rowell, 1974). An increase in erythrocyte, 2,3 DPG may be important in some patients with a limited cardiac output, but this is not found invariably.

In contrast, patients in whom O_2 extraction is poor have a higher cardiac output for a given O_2 intake. In present-day urban man, lack of exercise may lead to less than ideal distribution of blood to muscle and poor muscle O_2 extraction. If these changes exist with cardiac dysfunction, for example in ischemic heart disease, the impairment in exercise performance will be magnified, and the opposing effect

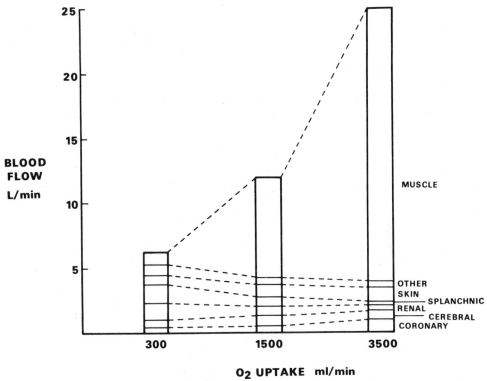

Figure 2–12   Regional distribution of blood flow during exercise. (From data given by Wade and Bishop, 1962.)

on the arteriovenous difference may lead to an erroneous interpretation of an exercise test in which cardiac frequency and O_2 intake alone are measured. In these situations a measurement of stroke volume to assess the central circulatory response and of blood lactate as an indication of peripheral O_2 uptake are required.

Intravascular Pressures

Systemic arterial blood pressure rises during exercise to levels around 200 mm Hg in maximal exercise. The rise in diastolic pressure is much less (to around 90 mm Hg), and mean arterial pressure increases from 90 mm Hg at rest to 140 mm Hg in maximal exercise (Holmgren, 1956). This modest increase contrasts with the fivefold or more increase in cardiac output, implying a considerable fall in systemic peripheral vascular resistance, presumably due to marked vasodilation in working muscle. Similarly, a considerable fall in pulmonary vascular resistance occurs during exercise; the rise in mean pulmonary artery pressure amounts to 15 mm Hg or less.

Although a limited stroke volume due to cardiac disease may lead to a low systemic arterial pressure, this is seldom observed because of the compensatory vasoconstriction. Occasionally a fall in arterial blood pressure may occur in patients with ischemic heart disease at the time that angina occurs. In systemic hypertension the rise in systemic pressure usually parallels the normal rise but remains above it (Sannerstedt et al, 1966), except during treatment with hypotensive agents, when blood pressure may fall to very low levels in exercise. The measurement of blood pressure is an important part of the exercise evaluation of any patient with suspected cardiac disease or hypertension.

The smaller capacity of the pulmonary vascular system makes it less able to adapt to an increase in vascular resistance. Patients with pulmonary vascular disease due to mitral stenosis, congenital septal defects, or pulmonary thromboembolism characteristically show marked increases in pulmonary artery pressure, sometimes to systemic levels, during exercise (Wilhelmsen et al, 1963).

Peripheral Vascular Changes

An increase in muscle perfusion occurs extremely rapidly at the onset of muscle contraction. The mechanism is uncertain but presumably is due to hypoxia and local changes in the concentration of lactic acid, ATP, and potassium (Barcroft, 1963; Rowell, 1974). Where blood flow to muscle is limited locally, as in peripheral atherosclerosis, exercise is often impeded by pain. Affected muscles exhibit a high oxygen extraction and increased lactic acid production.

In assessing the severity of the changes and in following the results of treatment it is important to choose a technique which ensures that the affected muscles are being exercised. Thus although cycle ergometry is a good way of studying the effects of major leg vessel obstruction, walking or calf-muscle exercise may be better for distal peripheral vascular disease.

Electrocardiographic Changes

Careful recording of the electrocardiograph has become a vital part of exercise testing. Changes in the ST segment are used as an important indicator of myocardial tissue hypoxia, occurring when myocardial oxygen demands exceed oxygen delivery; the criteria are reviewed later (p. 107). Tissue biopsy studies in experimental coronary occlusion have shown that the earliest biochemical indices of impaired myocardial O_2 delivery—reduced lactate extraction and potassium release—correlate well with local ST-segment changes recorded from the affected epicardium (Opie et al, 1973). The variation among different areas in the heart and the inconstant relationship between partial coronary arterial occlusion and an imbalance of O_2 supply and demand make it unlikely that any of the usual indicators—electrocardiographic, angiographic, or biochemical—will invariably identify myocardial ischemia. However, if care is taken with lead selection and recording (p. 77), electrocardiographic changes during exercise correlate well with other indices.

FITNESS

Several aspects of fitness have been alluded to already. Whether we define it in terms of the maximal $\dot{V}O_2$ per kg of body weight or more generally in terms of the capacity to enjoy moderate endurance activity without discomfort (Bannister, 1969), the term implies an optimal usage of the oxygen transport mechanisms, which allow exercising man to use his own stored energy resources and those of the environment to generate a power output without undue strain. The superior performance of an athlete is achieved through such optimal usage. Performance is dependent partly on attributes that are distributed throughout the healthy population such as variations due to sex; to body dimensions, which influence size of heart, lungs, and muscles; to age, mainly influencing maximal heart rate; and to hemoglobin content, influencing the oxygen-carrying capacity of the central circulation. Regular exercise leads to effective utilization of these attributes by increasing stroke volume, improving distribution of blood flow, and increasing muscle concentrations of glycogen and respiratory enzymes, among other general effects. The conventional measurement of fitness is maximal O_2 intake, which is usually expressed per kg of body weight (Max $\dot{V}O_2$/kg) in order to obtain a maximal power/weight ratio, which is a major determinant of endurance exercise. Often, however, this is not a convenient measurement to make in patients, and other measurements and relationships obtained during submaximal exercise may be used as indices of work capacity.

A practical approach to the measurement of fitness is to express changes in cardiac frequency and ventilation in terms of their capacity for adaptation predicted from such data as sex, age, and spirometry. Thus for a given increase in O_2 intake the fit person will use a smaller proportion of these capacities than an unfit subject (Spiro et al, 1974). The heart rate at a given power output or $\dot{V}O_2$ is lower in trained subjects than untrained, due to a larger stroke volume and slightly lower cardiac output, the arteriovenous oxygen difference being slightly higher at a given O_2 uptake. Thus the relationship of cardiac frequency to $\dot{V}O_2$ is an effective way of studying training in healthy subjects and in patients.

At the start of exercise, heart rate and cardiac output rapidly reach a steady level in trained subjects, which along with optimal blood flow distribution, leads to a reduced dependence on anaerobic metabolic pathways early in exercise. Consequently, blood lactate levels are lower than in untrained subjects. Trained subjects also may mobilize free fatty acids more rapidly (Havel et al, 1963). A low tissue respiratory quotient and minimal lactate production lead to a lower CO_2 output and less change in arterial pH, which in turn cause lower ventilation. The ventilatory demand is met primarily by an increase in tidal volume, resulting in a small V_D/V_T ratio and venous admixture.

However serious the effects of inactivity may be in otherwise healthy subjects, their importance becomes critical in patients with heart or lung disease, which may physically or psychologically limit activity. Because reserves of cardiac and ventilatory capacity are smaller, they are more readily encroached upon by inefficient usage. In the past, physicians have been guilty, through direct advice or implication, of unduly limiting their patients' activities and in so doing may have been responsible for a decline in their capacity for work. Training may be a valuable therapeutic tool when carefully used in these patients. In patients with coronary heart disease, training leads to a lower heart rate and to reduced myocardial oxygen requirements. Similar effects may be expected in patients with pulmonary disease; an improvement in the cardiovascular adaptation to exercise may induce a lower lactate production, lower CO_2 output, and thus smaller changes in blood PCO_2 and pH. These changes reduce the demand on a limited ventilatory capacity and make the most of any improvements in ventilation and gas exchange brought about by other therapeutic measures.

References

Andres, R., Cader, G. and Zierler, K. L.: Quantitatively minor role of carbohydrate in oxidative metabolism by skeletal muscle in intact man in basal state: measurements of oxygen and glucose uptake and carbon dioxide and lactate production in the forearm. J. Clin. Invest. *35*:671–682, 1956.

Åstrand, P. O., Hallback, I., Hedman, R. and Saltin, B.: Blood lactates after prolonged severe exercise. J. Appl. Physiol. 7:218, 1963.

Bannister, R.: The meaning of physical fitness. Proc. R. Soc. Med. *62*:1159, 1969.

Barcroft, H.: Circulation in skeletal muscle. *In* Hamilton, W. F. (ed.): Handbook of Physiology, vol. 2, Circulation Section II. Washington, D. C., American Physiological Society, 1963.

Bergström, J., Hermansen, L., Hultman, E. and Saltin, B.: Diet, muscle glycogen and physical performance. Acta Physiol. Scand. *71*:140-150, 1967.

Bevegård, S., Holmgren, A. and Jonsson, B.: The effect of body position on the circulation at rest and during exercise with special reference to the influence on the stroke volume. Acta Physiol. Scand. *49*:279-298, 1960.

Bevegård, S., Holmgren, A. and Jonsson, B.: Circulatory studies in well trained athletes at rest and during heavy exercise with special references to stroke volume and the influence of body position. Acta Physiol. Scand. *57*:26-56, 1963.

Böhr, C.: Ueber die Lungenathmung. Skand. Arch. Physiol. *2*:236–268, 1889.

Carlson, L. A., Ekelund, L.-G. and Fröberg, S. O.: Concentration of triglycerides, phospholipids and glycogen in skeletal muscle and of free fatty acids and B-Hydroxybutyric acid in blood in man in response to exercise. Eur. J. Clin. Invest. *1*:248–254, 1971.

Christensen, E. H., and Hansen, O.: Arbeitsfahigkeit and Erbanahoung. Skand. Arch. Physiol. *81*:160, 1939.

Clark, T. J. H., Freedman, S., Campbell, E. J. M. and Winn, R. R.: The ventilatory capacity of patients with chronic airways obstruction. Clin. Sci. *36*:307-316, 1969.

Cunningham, D. J. C.: Some quantitative aspects of the regulation of human respiration in exercise. Br. Med. Bull. *19*:25-30, 1963.

Edhag, O., and Zetterquist, S.: Peripheral circulatory adaptation to exercise in restricted cardiac output. Scand. J. Clin. Lab. Invest. *21*:123-135, 1968.

Edwards, R. H. T., Jones, D. A., Maunder, C., and Batra, G. J.: Needle biopsy for muscle chemistry. Lancet *1*:736–740, 1975.

Ekblom, B., Goldbarg, A. N. and Gullbring, B.: Response to exercise after blood loss and infusion. J. Appl. Physiol. *33*:175–180, 1972.

Ekblom, B., and Huot, R.: Response to submaximal and maximal exercise at different levels of carboxyhemoglobin. Acta Physiol. Scand. *86*:474-482, 1972.

Farhi, L. E.: Ventilation-perfusion relationship and its role in alveolar gas exchange. *In* C. G. Caro (ed.): Advances in Respiratory Physiology. London, Edward Arnold Publishers Ltd., 1966.

Felig, P., and Wahren, J.: Amino acid metabolism in exercising man. J. Clin. Invest. *50*:2703-2725, 1971.

Freedman, S.: Sustained maximum voluntary ventilation. Resp. Physiol. *8*:230–244, 1970.

Gollnick, P. D., Armstrong, G. R. B., Saltin, B., Saubert, C. W., Sembrowich, W. L. and Shepherd, R. E.: Effect of training on enzyme activity and fiber composition of human skeletal muscle. J. Appl. Physiol. *34*:107-111, 1973.

Gooch, A. S.: Exercise testing for detecting changes in cardiac rhythm and condition. Am. J. Cardiol. *30*:741-746, 1972.

Guz, A., Noble, M. I. M., Eisele, J. H. and Trenchard, D.: Experimental results of vagal block in cardiopulmonary disease. *In* Porter, R. (ed.): Breathing: Hering-Breuer Centenary Symposium. London: J. & A. Churchill, Ltd., 1970, p. 315.

Havel, R. J.: Some influences of the sympathetic nervous system and insulin on mobilization of fat from adipose tissue: studies of the turnover rates of free fatty acids and glycerol. Ann. N. Y. Acad. Sci. *131*:91-101, 1965.

Havel, R. J. Naimark, A. and Borchgrevink, C. F.: Turnover rate and oxidation of free fatty acids of blood plasma in man during exercise; studies during continuous infusion of palmitate-I-C^{14}. J. Clin. Invest. *42*:1054-1063, 1963.

Havel, R. J. Pernow, B. and Jones, N. L.: Uptake and release of free fatty acids and other metabolites in the legs of exercising men. J. Appl. Physiol. *23*:90-96, 1967.

Hermansen, L., and Osnes, J. B.: Blood and muscle pH after maximal exercise in man. J. Appl. Physiol. *32*:304-308, 1972.

Hesser, C. M., and Matell, G.: Effect of light and moderate exercise on alveolar-arterial O_2 tension difference in man. Acta Physiol. Scand. 63:247-256, 1965.

Holmgren, A.: Circulatory changes during muscular work in man. Scand. J. Clin. Lab. Invest. Suppl. 24, 1956.

Hultman, E., Bergström, J. and McLennan Anderson, N.: Breakdown and resynthesis of phosphorylcreatine and adenosine triphosphate in connection with muscular work in man. Scand. J. Clin. Lab. Invest. 19:56-66, 1967.

Jones, N. L.: Pulmonary gas exchange during exercise. M. D. Thesis, London Unversity, 1964.

Jones, N. L.: Pulmonary gas exchange during exercise in patients with chronic airway obstruction. Clin. Sci. 31:39-50, 1966.

Jones, N. L., and Goodwin, J. F.: Respiratory function in pulmonary thromboembolic disorders. Br. Med. J. 1:1089-1093, 1965.

Jones, N. L., and Haddon, R. W. T.: Effect of a meal on cardiopulmonary and metabolic changes during exercise. Can. J. Physiol. Pharm. 51:445-450, 1973.

Jones, N. L., Jones, G. and Edwards, R. H. T.: Exercise tolerance in chronic airway obstruction. Am. Rev.Resp. Dis. 103:477-491, 1971.

Jones, N. L., McHardy, G. J. R., Naimark, A. and Campbell, E. J. M.: Physiological dead space and alveolar-arterial gas pressure differences during exercise. Clin. Sci. 31:19-29, 1966.

Karlsson, J.: Lactate and phosphagen concentrations in working muscle of man. Acta Physiol. Scand. Suppl. 358, 1971.

Keul, J., Doll, E. and Keppler, D.: Energy Metabolism of Human Muscle: Medicine and Sport, vol. 7, Baltimore, University Park Press, 1971.

Lange-Anderson, K., Shephard, R. J., Denolin, H., Varnauskas, E. and Masironi, R.: Fundamentals of exercise testing. Geneva, World Health Organization, 1971.

Lehninger, A. L.: Biochemistry. New York, Worth Publishers Inc., 1970.

Lenfant, C., Ways, P., Aucutt, C. and Cruz, J.: Effect of chronic hypoxic hypoxia on the O_2-Hb dissociation curve and respiratory gas transport in man. Resp. Physiol. 7:7-29, 1969.

Levine, G., Housley, E., MacLeod, P. and Macklem, P. T.: Gas exchange abnormalities in mild bronchitis and asymptomatic asthma. New Engl. J. Med. 282:1277-1282, 1970.

McHardy, G. J. R.: Diffusing capacity and pulmonary gas exchange. Br. J. Dis. Chest 66:1-20, 1972.

Murray, J. M., and Weber, A.: The cooperative action of muscle proteins. Sci. Am. February 1974.

Needham, D.: Machina Carnis: the Biochemistry of Muscular Contraction in Its Historical Development. New York, Cambridge University Press, 1971.

Opie, L. H., Owen, P., Thomas, M. and Samson, R.: Coronary sinus lactate measurements in assessment of myocardial ischemia. Am. J. Cardiol. 32:295-305, 1973.

Parker, J. O.: The hemodynamic response to exercise in patients with healed myocardial infection without angina: with observations on the effects of nitroglycerin. Circulation 36:734-751, 1967.

Pernow, B., Havel, R. J. and Jennings, D. B.: The second wind phenomenon in McArdle's syndrome. Acta Med. Scand. (Suppl.) 472:294-307, 1967.

Pernow, B., Wahren, J, and Zetterquist, S.: Studies on the peripheral circulation and metabolism in man. IV. Oxygen utilization and lactate formation in the legs of healthy young men during strenuous exercise. Acta Physiol. Scand. 64:289-298, 1965.

Piiper, J.: Measurement of the gas-exchanging function of the lung. Revision of concepts, quantities and units in gas-exchange physiology. Proc. Roy. Soc. Med. 66:971-980, 1973.

Rebuck, A. S., Jones, N. L. and Campbell, E. J. M.: Ventilatory response to exercise and to CO_2 rebreathing in normal subjects. Clin. Sci. 43:861-867, 1973.

Rebuck, A. S., Jones, N. L. and Pengelly, L. D.: Tidal volume response to exercise in normal subjects with inspiratory elastic loading and in patients with stiff lungs. Bull. Physio-Path. Resp. 9:1266, 1973.

Redwood, D. R., Rosing, D. R. and Epstein, S. E.: Circulatory and symptomatic effects of physical training in patients with coronary-artery disease and angina pectoris. New Engl. J. Med. 286:959-991, 1972.

Riley, R. L., and Cournand, A.: "Ideal" alveolar air and the analysis of ventilation perfusion relationships in the lungs. J. Appl. Physiol. 1:825-847, 1949.

Riley, R. L., and Cournand, A.: Analysis of factors affecting partial pressures of oxygen and carbon dioxide in gas and blood of lungs: theory. J. Appl. Physiol. 4:77-101, 1951.

Rowell, L. B.: Human cardiovascular adjustments to exercise and thermal stress. Physiol. Rev. 54:75-159, 1974.

Saltin, B., Blomquist, B., Mitchell, J. H., Johnson, R. L., Wildenthal, K. and Chapman, C. B.: Response to submaximal and maximal exercise after bed rest and training. Circulation 38; Suppl. 7, 1968.

Sannerstedt, R., Schroder, G. and Werkö, L.: Clinical pharmacology and short-term treatment. Haemodynamic analysis of some principles applied in the treatment of arterial hypertension. Antihypertensive Therapy Principles & Practice 268-281, 1966.

Segel, N., Hudson, W. A., Harris, P. and Bishop, J. M.: The circulatory effects of electrically induced changes in ventricular rate at rest and during exercise in complete heart block. J. Clin. Invest. 43:1541-1550, 1964.

Shapell, S. D., Murray, J. A., Nasser, M. G., Wills, R. E., Torrance, J. D. and Lenfant, C. J. M.: Acute change in hemoglobin affinity for oxygen during angina pectoris. New Engl. J. Med. 282:1219-1224, 1970.

Shephard, R. J.: Oxygen cost of breathing during vigorous exercise. Quart. J. Exp. Physiol. 51:336-350, 1966.

Sjöstrand, T.: Functional capacity and exercise tolerance in patients with impaired cardiovascular function. In Gordon, B. L. (ed.): Clinical Cardiopulmonary Physiology. New York, Grune & Stratten, Inc., 1960.

Sonnenblick, E. H., Braunwald, E., Williams, J. F. and Glick, G.: Effects of exercise on myocardial force-velocity relations in intact unanesthetized man: relative roles of changes in heart rate, sympathetic activity, and ventricular dimensions. J. Clin. Invest. 44:2051-2062, 1965.

Spiro, S. G., Juniper, E., Bowman, P. and Edwards, R. H. T.: An increasing work rate for assessing the physiological strain of submaximal exercise. Clin. Sci. and Molecular Med. 46:191-206, 1974.

Vedin, J. A., Wilhelmsson, C. E., Wilhelmsen, L., Bjure, J. and Ekström-Jodal, B.: Relation of resting and exercise-induced ischemic manifestations and to coronary risk factors. Am. J. Cardiol. 30:25-31, 1972.

Wade, O. L., and Bishop, J. M.: Cardiac Output and Regional Blood Flow. (Blackwell Scientific Pubns.) Philadelphia, F. A. Davis Co., 1962.

Werkö, L.: Mitral Valvular Disease. Haemodynamic Studies of the Consequences for the Circulation. Baltimore, Williams & Wilkens Co., 1964.

Young, D. R., Shapira, J., Forrest, R., Adachi, R. R., Lim, R. and Pelligra, R.: Model for evaluation of fatty acid metabolism for man during prolonged exercise. J. Appl. Physiol. 23:716-725, 1967.

West, J. B.: Distribution of gas and blood in the normal lung. Br. Med. Bull. 19:53-58, 1963.

Wilhemsen, L., Selander, S., Söderholm, B., Paulin, S., Varnauskas, E. and Werkö, L.: Recurrent pulmonary embolism. Medicine 42:335-355, 1963.

Wilkie, D. R.: Man as a source of mechanical power. Ergonomics 3:1-18, 1960.

Chapter Three

APPROACHES TO EXERCISE TESTING

In developing an exercise testing facility, several alternative methods and procedures exist, and decisions have to be made regarding the following:

1. Type of exercise.
2. Duration and intensity of exercise.
3. Observations to be made.

The choices will depend on the types of patient to be studied and the complexity and kind of information required. This chapter will outline the available methods and the information that can be obtained from a variety of procedures. The procedures vary widely in complexity—some are simple and do not require expensive equipment, but many are intricate and demand considerable outlay in terms of equipment and personnel. A complex procedure may generate more measurements than a simple one but may add little to the assessment of certain patients. For example, if the clinical problem is that of a cardiac murmur in an adolescent, it is usually possible to answer the question, "Is there impaired cardiac function," by a simple test that occupies the patient and the laboratory for less than 30 minutes and which does not involve blood vessel catheterization. The cardiac catheterization laboratory may then be used to answer difficult problems which require hemodynamic measurements for their solution. Over the past decade we have come to rely on a series of procedures that utilize increasing levels or "stages" of complexity and derived information; we have found that this approach encourages an economical use of resources. These stages will be described in principle later in this chapter, and details are given in Chapter 5.

TYPES OF EXERCISE USED FOR TESTING

In most situations the aim of testing is to exercise large muscle groups in order to stress muscle metabolism and the cardiovascular and respiratory systems. Special requirements for individual limbs or muscle groups will not be considered here. For the purpose of description, three broad areas can be recognized:

1. Everyday exercise.
2. Poorly standardized tests using steps or stairs.
3. Standardized tests using treadmills and cycle ergometers.

Everyday Exercise

At their simplest, exercise tests are an extension of clinical examination. They entail the observation of the patient walking along a corridor or up one or more flights of stairs and measurement of the patient's frequency of breathing and heart rate. When it is important to know the demands that occur during everyday activities, such as at work in industry, telemetry or lightweight portable recording systems (Weiner and Lourie, 1969; Holter, 1961) are used to measure heart rate; measurements of ventilation and oxygen intake can be made using portable equipment such as the Kofranyi-Michaelis respirometer (Müller and Franz, 1952) or the Wolff IMP (Wolff, 1958). For a further discussion of energy demands of everyday activity, the reader is referred to the comprehensive review of Durnin and Passmore (1968).

Steps

For more formal testing, steps are not only trouble-free but can be used in a clinic or examining room where space is limited. Variations in work rate can be achieved by altering the step height or the frequency of stepping (Nagle et al, 1965), but precise measurement of the power developed is impossible owing to the difficulty in calculating the work performed in stepping off the step. Very high work rates cannot be developed because the step height and rate of stepping have to be uncomfortably large. Shephard (1966), in reviewing several methods, suggest a constant step height and variable stepping rate. Gupta et al (1973) have described a progressive step test in which both step height and rate are varied. In the most commonly used step test described by Master and Rosenfield (1967) for diagnosis of myocardial ischemia, the electrocardiogram is recorded before and after exercise. Additional information is obtained by recording the electrocardiogram continuously so that changes in heart rate, rhythm, and the electrocardiogram complex can be followed closely during the exercise. The continual movement during a step test makes it difficult to collect expired gas or to sample blood, but a measure of ventilation may be obtained by using a Wright anemometer (Wright, 1958), or by having the patient hold a light breathing valve connected to a gas meter by flexible wide bore tubing (Gupta et al, 1973).

The information obtainable from these tests is limited but may be of considerable help in the office assessment of patients and in field studies where a limited amount of equipment can be used.

Treadmills and Cycles

Measurement of several physiological variables requires a treadmill or cycle ergometer, which enable an accurately known power output to be used.

The *treadmill* is preferred by many because walking is a universal activity, whereas few adults ride bicycles, so that the exercise is considered to be more appropriate to the patient's daily life. Although the "staged" exercise testing approach described below may be applied with treadmill exercise, there are several disadvantages. It is difficult to set a desired workload, because this depends on the weight of the patient, the speed, and the grade of incline; in addition, body lift on the treadmill is variable and unmeasurable. Should the patient be unable to meet the demand, there is a danger of falling; the treadmill cannot be stopped instantly or safely in this situation. Furthermore, treadmills are bulky, expensive, and noisy in operation, and many patients find that walking rapidly with the head attached to a mouthpiece for expired gas collection is less comfortable than performing on a cycle ergometer.

With *cycle ergometers* a workload can be changed quickly and easily, and a predictable metabolic response is obtained as long as the ergometer is accurately calibrated. If the patient becomes distressed and ceases pedaling, work stops instantly. In average subjects cycling does not produce as high a maximum oxygen uptake as a treadmill, but ventilation and lactate production are slightly higher

(Shephard et al, 1968). These variations are due to the different muscle groups used, and although they may be important in comparing populations, they are not significant in clinical practice. Discomfort in the leg muscles is more common on a cycle ergometer than on a treadmill but can be reduced by proper positioning of the patient. Many cycles can be used with the subject in either an erect or supine position, the latter being an advantage if cardiac catheterization measurements are to be made.

INTENSITY AND DURATION OF TESTS

Ideally, patients should be studied at several power outputs up to their maximum, and each output should be maintained long enough for a "steady state" to be reached in O_2 intake and the cardiorespiratory adaptations. However, in most patients this ideal cannot, or should not, be attempted as it may lead to unnecessary discomfort or risk; a compromise has to be reached between the number and intensity of power outputs and the necessity for a steady state. If measurements are required at several power outputs to a maximum level or close to it, the steady state may have to be sacrificed. However, if measurements requiring a steady state are essential, two or three power outputs are studied up to 60 to 80 per cent of the subject's maximum; these power outputs may then be sustained long enough for a steady state to be reached.

These considerations led us to adopt two forms of exercise test. In the first, power output is increased every minute, and constant values for oxygen intake ($\dot{V}O_2$) are not reached; thus measurements are made in an "unsteady state." In the second form of test, power output is constant long enough for most variables to reach relatively constant steady-state values. Rapid increases in $\dot{V}O_2$ and $\dot{V}CO_2$ occur in the first 2 to 4 minutes after an increase in workload, but changes thereafter are small (Ekelund, 1967). Thus after 4 to 5 minutes' exercise at a constant work rate, a steady state will have been maintained long enough for measurements of cardiac output and pulmonary gas exchange to be valid.

Progressive Multistage Test (Stage 1)

In this test the power output is increased by a constant amount at the end of each minute. With a cycle ergometer, the work rate is raised by 100 kpm/min (16 w) every minute. On a treadmill, increases in work rate can be imposed by increases of 2 per cent in incline at a constant speed of 80 m/min (3 mph) (Fox et al, 1971). The test continues to the patient's maximum or until stopped by the operator either because a target power output or cardiac frequency has been reached or because of untoward symptoms or signs (p. 84). Established or suspected ischemic heart disease requires caution: in the interests of safety the American Heart Association has recommended than an "age related target heart rate" of 85 per cent of the maximum predicted from the patient's age should not be exceeded (p. 35). However, accuracy in predicting maximum cardiac frequency is only ± 20 beats/min. Furthermore, there is increasing evidence that one of the manifestations of myocardial disease is an inability to increase cardiac frequency normally, with a maximum frequency which may be substantially lower than predicted. In this situation the "target heart rate" may be unrealistically high. Thus although 85 per cent of the predicted maximum cardiac frequency should generally not be exceeded in patients with suspected myocardial ischemia, it is important to have accurate monitoring facilities, trained staff, and a laboratory discipline with established criteria for stopping a test. Such facilities will allow most patients to be taken to a symptom-limited maximum with safety.

Constant Power Output Steady State Tests
(Stages 2, 3, and 4)

In these tests, measurements are made in a *steady state* during exercise at two or more submaximal power outputs, ideally chosen using the results from a Stage 1 test. Usually power outputs corresponding to 1/3 and 2/3 of the highest power output completed in the Stage 1 procedure are chosen; if the latter exceeds 900 kpm/min (150 w), three power outputs may be chosen corresponding to 1/4, 1/2, and 3/4 of the maximum. If information from a Stage 1 test is unavailable, two or three power outputs are chosen according to the patient's symptoms or the predicted cardiac frequency response. Each power output is sustained for at least two minutes after measurements reveal a steady state of cardiac frequency, O_2 intake, and CO_2 output, to allow for expired gas collection, rebreathing, or blood sampling, as required. This means that each power output is sustained for 5 to 8 minutes, as in the exercise testing procedure widely used in Scandinavia (Sjöstrand, 1960).

Successive increases in power output may be made continuously; however, where significant cardiac disease is suspected it is probably wise to separate each power output by a two-minute period of loadless pedaling, during which time the electrocardiograph is recorded and the patient's symptoms carefully assessed.

OBSERVATIONS MADE DURING EXERCISE TESTS

The description of the normal responses to exercise and their alteration in a wide variety of conditions given in Chapter 2 will have suggested a large number of measurements that could be of value in the assessment of patients. Many would argue that all the measurements within the laboratory's capability should be made in all patients, but we believe this is an unrealistic approach if the maximum benefit from exercise testing is to be obtained in the maximum number of patients. Parallels could be drawn from other clinical investigations; for example, there is little point in applying a vast array of hematological techniques to a problem which can be answered by a blood smear. These are the reasons for adopting the following series of testing procedures involving measurements of increasing complexity.

Stage 1: heart rate and ventilation, preferably with O_2 intake and CO_2 output; blood pressure; electrocardiograph.
Stage 2: adds O_2 intake, CO_2 output, and the PCO_2 of mixed expired gas and mixed venous blood.
Stage 3: adds blood gases, pH, and lactate.
Stage 4: adds right heart pressures.

The choice of measurements is dictated by physiological as well as technical and logistic considerations. The results are interpreted in relation to the power output recorded from the settings on the cycle ergometer or treadmill. It should be emphasized that wherever possible, variables should be related to O_2 intake rather than to mechanical power output: this allows values obtained from a variety of exercise protocols to be compared directly. For example, heart rate and ventilation measurements obtained in a Stage 1 test are closely comparable at a given O_2 intake to those obtained in a steady state (Stage 2). Although the interpretation of results will be left for a later chapter, the type of information obtained from each of these stages will be reviewed briefly here.

Stage 1

In this test, measurements of cardiac frequency and ventilation (and blood pressure if necessary) are made at several power outputs, which are maintained for a minute each, the measurements being made during the last 15 seconds of each minute. If mixed expired gas concentrations are measured as well, $\dot{V}O_2$ and $\dot{V}CO_2$ can be calculated; in this way the variables can be related to O_2 intake and CO_2 output, simplifying interpretation and comparison between tests. The electrocardiograph is recorded before the test, at the end of each minute, and after 1, 2, and 5 minutes of recovery — longer if an abnormality occurs.

The results are examined in terms of the cardiac frequency response to the power output or $\dot{V}O_2$ and the ventilatory response to power output or $\dot{V}CO_2$. Breathing frequency and tidal volume are measured, and the evolution of the breathing pattern is examined over a wide range of ventilation. If the results are examined in relation to each other, interpretation becomes more precise, and there is less need for measurements to be made in a steady state. Maximum $\dot{V}O_2$ may be either directly measured or calculated from submaximal values. Blood lactate may be measured in a sample of blood taken in the first two minutes of recovery.

The advantages of this procedure are that measurements are made at several workloads; the measurements are simple, requiring only one observer; and the whole procedure takes less than 20 minutes.

Stage 2

Although the information obtained from a Stage 1 test may allow the possibility of significant heart or lung disease to be excluded, an abnormal response may be difficult to interpret in terms of changes in cardiac output and stroke volume, alveolar ventilation and pulmonary gas exchange, and metabolism. However, it is possible to obtain estimates, or to establish useful limits for these variables, using a bloodless technique (Jones, 1967). The approach employs mathematical analysis of the variables to obtain information regarding a series of linked functions. The relationships are reviewed briefly here so that the logic behind the measurements may be appreciated. They will be explored more fully in Chapter 10 with the use of some examples.

1. The CO_2 transport system may be considered as starting in the tissues with the production of CO_2 from aerobic metabolism of carbohydrate and fat. In addition, CO_2 will be evolved from the reaction of lactic acid with tissue fluid bicarbonate, which generates carbonic acid. Most of the CO_2 produced from these two sources will be excreted in expired gas, but some CO_2 may ac-

cumulate in body stores, leading to an increase in tissue P_{CO_2}. Thus a balance equation may be constructed for CO_2 as follows:

(a) Total CO_2 output = (b) CO_2 from aerobic metabolism ± (c) changes in CO_2 stores + (d) CO_2 from lactate.

In this equation (a) is measured, (b) is estimated from the O_2 intake, and (c) is estimated from changes in mixed venous P_{CO_2}; (d) may then be derived, yielding an indirect estimate of lactate accumulation (Clode and Campbell, 1969).

2. Fick's principle applied to CO_2 is expressed as follows:

$$\text{Cardiac output} = \frac{CO_2 \text{ output}}{\text{veno-arterial } CO_2 \text{ difference}}$$

$$\dot{Q}_t = \frac{\dot{V}_{CO_2}}{C_{\bar{v}}CO_2 - C_aCO_2}$$

or

$$\dot{Q}_t = \frac{\dot{V}_{CO_2}}{f(P_{\bar{v}}CO_2 - P_aCO_2)}$$

where f is a function of the blood CO_2 dissociation curve.

3. Alveolar ventilation ($\dot{V}_A$) determines the arterial P_{CO_2}.

$$P_aCO_2 = \frac{\dot{V}_{CO_2} \times 0.863}{\dot{V}_A}$$

4. The dead space:tidal volume ratio determines the mixed expired P_{CO_2} for a given P_aCO_2.

$$V_D/V_T = \frac{P_aCO_2 - P_ECO_2}{P_aCO_2}$$

From (2), (3), and (4) above it can be seen that at a given CO_2 output the mixed venous P_{CO_2} and mixed expired P_{CO_2} are governed by cardiac output, alveolar ventilation, and the V_D/V_T ratio, all of which are linked to the arterial P_{CO_2}.

The mixed venous to arterial P_{CO_2} difference is dependent on the cardiac output, and the arterial to mixed expired P_{CO_2} difference is dependent on the V_D/V_T ratio. Thus a low cardiac output or high

V_D/V_T ratio tends to increase the difference between mixed venous P_{CO_2} and mixed expired P_{CO_2}, from which it is possible to place limits on cardiac output and the V_D/V_T ratio without measuring arterial P_{CO_2}. This provides quantitative information regarding cardiac output and pulmonary response to exercise without taking blood. As outlined in (1) above, lactate accumulation may be estimated.

In order to apply this analysis, the following measurements are made during a steady state: CO_2 output, O_2 intake, mixed expired P_{CO_2}, and mixed venous P_{CO_2}. Other observations such as arterial blood pressure and the electrocardiograph are also made.

The bloodless nature of this test makes it relatively simple for subject and operator, and the total time taken is less than 40 minutes.

Stage 3

This procedure adds arterial blood sampling (or some acceptable alternative) to the Stage 2 measurements. In addition to the measurement of P_aCO_2 (from which $\dot{Q}_t$, $\dot{V}_A$, and V_D/V_T are calculated), lactate, arterial pH, and P_{O_2} are measured, enabling the alveolar-arterial P_{O_2} difference and venous admixture to be calculated. Almost all of the relationships reviewed in Chapter 2 can be examined fully. Thus additional information is obtained but at a cost of increased numbers of assistants as well as more time, an average of 90 minutes being needed. Although on occasion it may be obvious that Stage 3 information is required for the adequate assessment of a patient, it is usually better to perform a Stage 1 or Stage 2 test first and proceed to Stage 3 on another occasion if required. In this way the power outputs to be studied in a Stage 3 test can be correctly chosen. In addition, the total experience of arterial puncture and an exercise test may be too much for some patients to bear with equanimity unless they have been prepared by a preceding bloodless test.

An acceptable compromise, either as an addition to the Stage 2 or as a substitute for the Stage 3, may be achieved by sampling arterialized capillary blood, if facilities exist for the measurement of blood gases and pH in small blood samples.

Stage 4

This procedure adds right heart catheterization by float catheter (Swan-Ganz) to the Stage 3 test and is used only where right heart pressures are required.

CONCLUSION

Our experience has been that for the majority of patients referred for exercise testing, an adequate assessment is obtained from Stage 1 or Stage 2 tests. These procedures have the advantage of being technically simple enough to establish as a laboratory routine and are recommended for any laboratory in which clinical exercise testing is being instituted. They require a modest initial outlay in terms of equipment and staff, and development of other facilities may be left to a later stage after experience has been gained and the need established.

References

Clode, M., and Campbell, E. J. M.: The relationship between gas exchange and changes in blood lactate concentrations during exercise. Clin. Sci. 37:263–272, 1969.

Durnin, J. V. G. A., and Passmore, R.: Energy, Work and Leisure. London, William Heinemann Ltd., 1968.

Ekelund, L.-G.: Circulatory and respiratory adaptation during prolonged exercise of moderate intensity in the sitting position. Acta Physiol. Scand. 69:327–340, 1967.

Fox, S. M., Naughton, J. P. and Haskell, W. L.: Physical activity and the prevention of coronary heart disease. Ann. Clin. Res. 3:404, 1971.

Gupta, S. A., Fletcher, C. M. and Edwards, R. H. T.: Progressive exercise step test. J. Assoc. Physicians India 21:555–564, 1973.

Holter, N. L.: New method for heart studies. Science 134:1214–1220, 1961.

Jones, N. L.: Exercise testing. Br. J. Dis. Chest 61:169–189, 1967.

Master, A. M., and Rosenfeld, I.: Exercise electrocardiography as an estimation of cardiac function. Dis. Chest 51:347–382, 1967.

Müller, E. A., and Franz, H.: Energieverbrauchsmessungen bei beruflicher Arbeit mit einer verbesserten Respirations-Gesuhr. Int. Z. Angew. Physiol. 14:499–504, 1952.

Nagle, F. J., Blake, B. and Naughton, J. F.: Gradational step tests for assessing work capacity. J. Appl. Physiol. 20:745–748, 1965.

Shephard, R. J.: The relative merits of the step test, bicycle ergometer and treadmill in the assessment of cardio-respiratory fitness. Int. Z. Angew. Physiol. 23:219–230, 1966.

Shephard, R. J., Allen, C., Benade, A. J. S., Davies, C. T. M., DiPrampero, P. E., Hedman, R., Merriman, J. E., Myhre, K. and Simmons, R.: Standardization of submaximal exercise tests. Bull. WHO 38:765–775, 1968.

Sjöstrand, T.: Functional capacity and exercise tolerance in patients with impaired cardiovascular function. In Gordon, B. L. (ed.): Clinical Cardiopulmonary Physiology. New York, Grune & Stratton, Inc., 1960, pp. 201–219.

Weiner, J. S., and Lourie, J. A.: Human Biology. A Guide to Field Methods. (Blackwell Scientific Pubns.) Philadelphia, F. A. Davis Co., 1969.

Wolff, H. S.: The integrating pneumotachograph: a new instrument for the measurement of energy expenditure by indirect calorimetry. Quart. J. Exp. Physiol. 43:270–283, 1958.

Wright, B. M.: A respiratory anemometer. J. Physiol. (London) 127:25, 1958.

Chapter Four

MIXED VENOUS Pco$_2$ AND THE MEASUREMENT OF CARDIAC OUTPUT

In the Stage 2 and 3 tests described in Chapter 3, mixed venous Pco$_2$ is used during exercise for the measurement of cardiac output (Stage 3) or for establishing limits for cardiac output and the V_D/V_T ratio (Stage 2). In this chapter we will review the reasons for our reliance on this method, and the principles involved in the measurement, leaving the technical details for a later chapter.

Several methods are well established for the measurement of cardiac output, but for various reasons they are difficult to apply in routine exercise testing.

THE DIRECT FICK METHOD

The standard by which other methods are usually judged is the *direct Fick method*, in which oxygen content is measured in samples of arterial and mixed venous blood obtained simultaneously while expired gas is collected. Cardiac output is then calculated from the following equation:

$$\text{Cardiac output} = \frac{\text{oxygen uptake}}{\text{arteriovenous oxygen content difference}}$$

that is,

$$\dot{Q}_t = \frac{\dot{V}o_2}{C_a o_2 - C_{\bar{v}} o_2}$$

For greatest accuracy, the mixed venous blood should be obtained from the pulmonary artery, but the need for pulmonary arterial catheterization severely restricts the use of this method.

INDICATOR DILUTION TECHNIQUE

In the *indicator dilution* technique a dye is injected as a bolus into the right side of the central circulation, and blood flow is derived from the resulting dilution curve obtained by passing arterial blood through a densitometer. Under ideal conditions the results obtained are within ± 10 per cent of values obtained with the direct Fick method (Holmgren and Pernow, 1959). However, both arterial and venous catheterization are required.

Dye may be injected in a peripheral vein and the dilution curve obtained from a cuvette attached to the ear lobe. Unfortunately, this technique is not generally applicable during exercise, due to the quality of the dilution curve.

FOREIGN GAS METHODS

In the *foreign gas* methods a soluble gas such as acetylene or nitrous oxide is inspired, and the cardiac output is calculated from the amount taken up in the lungs, its solubility, and the mean alveolar gas concentration. For many years the acetylene technique (Grollman, 1929) was the most widely used method for measuring cardiac output, but it was virtually abandoned when the direct Fick method was introduced. However, several foreign-gas methods have regained popularity in exercise physiology, including acetylene (Pugh, 1964) and nitrous oxide (Becklake et al, 1962; Rigatto, 1967; Ayotte et al, 1970). Although no blood samples are needed, difficulty may be experienced in obtaining an accurate estimate of mean alveolar concentration, particularly in many patients with lung disease where there is poor mixing of gases in the lungs.

INDIRECT FICK METHODS

The term "indirect" Fick is used to describe methods in which the mixed venous blood oxygen or carbon dioxide contents are derived from their partial pressure in the gas phase, with the lungs acting as a tonometer, rather than in the directly sampled mixed venous blood. The approach was popular at the beginning of the century

(Plesch, 1909) but later fell into disfavor, mainly because sufficient accuracy could not be obtained with the equipment available at the time. The renaissance of the method is attributable to two factors: first, the advent of rapid physical analyzers for accurate detection and measurement of the equilibrium of P_{CO_2} between alveolar gas and mixed venous blood, and secondly, the appreciation that during exercise the increased venoarterial O_2 and CO_2 pressure differences lead to greater precision in the measurement of cardiac output.

Because indirect methods do not require cardiac catheterization, there are obvious advantages in routine exercise testing. Although methods are established for measuring mixed venous O_2 as well as CO_2, the former cannot be recommended for routine exercise testing, due to the transient severe hypoxemia which occurs during the procedure (Denison et al, 1971).

Two approaches have been used for the measurement of the mixed venous P_{CO_2} during exercise.

1. *Rebreathing from a bag containing a low concentration of carbon dioxide.* When a bag containing a low percentage of carbon dioxide in oxygen is rebreathed, the P_{CO_2} rises exponentially towards the pulmonary arterial (mixed venous) P_{CO_2}. Mixed venous P_{CO_2} is obtained by extrapolating the end expiratory P_{CO_2} values before recirculation to a point where the P_{CO_2} equals that of the preceding breath: this is the mixed venous P_{CO_2} (Defares, 1958; Jernérus et al, 1963). However, the changes between succeeding breaths are generally small, and variation results in a large potential error in the extrapolated value. This may be the reason for poor repeatability of results; for example, Godfrey and Wolf (1972) reported a coefficient of variation of nearly 6 per cent in repeated studies in healthy subjects, far greater than for the equilibrium method described below (1.1 per cent). In addition, changes in breathing pattern and gas mixing in the lungs will lead to greater errors in patients with lung disease.

2. *Equilibration method, using a bag containing a high concentration of carbon dioxide in oxygen.* If a subject rebreathes from a bag containing gas at a P_{CO_2} sufficiently higher than mixed venous P_{CO_2}, the gas in the bag mixes with the alveolar gas, and CO_2 is removed by pulmonary capillary blood until an equilibrium occurs between the P_{CO_2} in the bag, alveolar gas, and pulmonary capillary blood. The equilibrium indicates the lack of net movement of CO_2 and that alveolar P_{CO_2} equals the P_{CO_2} of oxygenated mixed venous blood. The patterns of CO_2 during rebreathing and the criteria for equilibration are discussed more fully in a later chapter (p. 95).

An objection to the equilibration method is that the high P_{CO_2} or the increased frequency of breathing affect the mixed venous P_{CO_2}, so that the value obtained in a subsequent rebreathing will be in error. However, we have been unable to detect changes in heart rate or pulmonary hemodynamics during rebreathing. The effect of CO_2 accumulation is avoided by allowing 30 seconds to elapse before repeating the procedure. With this precaution, mixed venous PCO$_2$ is reproducible to ± 2 mm Hg.

Satisfactory equilibration patterns can be obtained even in patients with severe ventilation-perfusion disturbances in the lungs, if the bag volume and CO_2 concentration are carefully chosen. Although equilibration between the gas in the rebreathing bag and poorly ventilated areas may be slow, the PCO$_2$ in these areas will be close to mixed venous values, thus minimizing any effect they might have on the attainment of equilibrium. We have used this method extensively during the past ten years and found it to be a simple and effective technique which can be used in a wide variety of patients.

VALIDITY OF RESULTS

If the mixed venous and arterial PCO$_2$ are known, the venoarterial CO_2 content difference may be derived using a standard CO_2 dissociation curve. Appropriate corrections are made for changes in hemoglobin and arterial O_2 desaturation, both factors affecting the relationship of CO_2 pressure to content in whole blood. Cardiac output is then calculated from the venoarterial CO_2 content difference and CO_2 output using Fick's principle.

When the equilibration method was first used, it was found that the values for cardiac output obtained during exercise on a cycle ergometer were lower than the estimates for cardiac output using dye dilution or the direct Fick (oxygen) method (Jones et al, 1967). At high work rates (O_2 intake 2.5 L/min or above) the differences amounted to as much as 10 per cent, suggesting that the mixed venous PCO$_2$ obtained by rebreathing was too high. This problem was investigated by comparing the PCO$_2$ in the gas phase during a rebreathing equilibrium with the PCO$_2$ in the blood sampled from the pulmonary artery (Denison et al, 1969) and from a systemic artery (Jones et al, 1967). In both studies the PCO$_2$ in the gas phase was found to be higher than the PCO$_2$ in the blood. This difference is of interest in its own right because it indicates incomplete CO_2 equilibration within blood or across the alveolar-capillary membrane (Jones et al, 1969). Until the mechanisms have been elucidated, some doubt will exist regarding the accuracy of estimates of venous CO_2 content from the rebreathing PCO$_2$ values. However, studies in a wide variety of situations have shown that a correction may be applied to the equilibrium P_{CO_2} to obtain a P_{CO_2} which should accurately reflect mixed venous CO_2 content. The details of this correction are given in Appendix 3. If the method described in Chapter 6 is followed, mixed venous P_{CO_2} is estimated to within ± 2 mm Hg.

An accurate measure of cardiac output also depends on the accuracy of arterial P_{CO_2} measurement. Rigorously calibrated, the CO_2 electrode will measure arterial P_{CO_2} to within ± 1 mm Hg. Alternatively, capillary blood or arterialized venous blood may be used, as long as simple rules are observed to ensure adequate arterialization. Arterial P_{CO_2} may also be estimated from the end tidal P_{CO_2} with an accuracy of ± 2 mm Hg, as long as the subject does not show evidence of poor gas distribution in the lungs. These methods are detailed in a later chapter.

The relative accuracy of measurements of cardiac output using this method increases with increasing power output, because accuracy is dependent largely on the P_{CO_2} analyses, and the venoarterial CO_2 difference increases with increasing exercise. This contrasts with some other methods, for example dye dilution, in which the analysis becomes more prone to error at high cardiac outputs.

As with any method proposed for the measurement of cardiac output in a routine exercise laboratory, the accuracy of the rebreathing CO_2 method is difficult to establish, and comparative studies with other methods under ideal conditions with fully co-operative subjects and a skilled team may not be applied uncritically to everyday practice. Long experience, however, has demonstrated its value in the assessment of patients. It is simple to use, can be repeated often, and has great advantages in children and in adult patients in whom the clinical problem does not warrant cardiac catheterization. Accuracy depends on attention to technical details, which are given in Chapter 6.

References

Ayotte, B., Seymour, J. and McIlroy, M.: A new method for measurement of cardiac output with nitrous oxide. J. Appl. Physiol. 28:863–866, 1970.

Becklake, M. R., Varvis, C. J., Pengelly, L. D., Kenning, S., McGregor, M. and Bates, D. V.: Measurement of pulmonary blood flow during exercise using nitrous oxide. J. Appl. Physiol. 17:579–586, 1962.

Defares, J. G.: Determination of $P\bar{v}CO_2$ from the exponential CO_2 rise during rebreathing. J. Appl. Physiol. 13:159–164, 1958.

Denison, D., Edwards, R. H. T., Jones, G. and Pope, H.: Direct and rebreathing estimates of the O_2 and CO_2 pressures in mixed venous blood. Resp. Physiol. 7:326–334, 1969.

Denison, D., Edwards, R. H. T., Jones, G. and Pope, H.: Estimates of the CO_2 pressures in systemic arterial blood during rebreathing on exercise. Resp. Physiol. *11*:186–196, 1971.

Godfrey, S., and Wolf, E.: An evaluation of rebreathing methods for measuring mixed venous Pco_2 during exercise. Clin. Sci. *42*:345–353, 1972.

Grollman, A.: The determination of the cardiac output of man by the use of acetylene. Am. J. Physiol. *88*:432–445, 1929.

Holmgren, A., and Pernow, B.: Spectrophotometric measurement of oxygen saturation of blood in the determination of cardiac output. A comparison with the Van Slyke method. Scand. J. Clin. Lab. Invest. *11*:143–149, 1959.

Jernérus, R., Lundin, G., and Thomson, D.: Cardiac output in healthy subjects determined with a CO_2 rebreathing method. Acta Physiol. Scand. *59*:390–399, 1963.

Jones, N. L., Campbell, E. J. M., Edwards, R. H. T. and Wilkoff, G.: Alveolar to blood Pco_2 difference during rebreathing in exercise. J. Appl. Physiol. *27*:356–360, 1969.

Jones, N. L., Campbell, E. J. M., McHardy, G. J. R., Higgs, B. E. and Clode, M.: The estimation of carbon dioxide pressure of mixed venous blood during exercise. Clin. Sci. *32*:311–327, 1967.

Plesch, J.: Hamodynamische studien. A Exp. Path. Therap. *6*:380–618, 1909.

Pugh, L. G. C. E.: Cardiac output in muscular exercise at 5,800 m (19,000 ft.). J. Appl. Physiol. *19*:441–447, 1964.

Rigatto, M.: Mass spectrometry in the study of the pulmonary circulation. Bull. Physiopathol. Resp. *3*:473–486, 1967.

Chapter Five

EQUIPMENT

This chapter is intended for the reader who wants to know what equipment is needed for exercise testing. It is not an exhaustive review; we have limited ourselves to general observations because the range of some items of equipment is now so large that we are unable to provide a "consumers' guide" of instruments from all sources. However, the manufacturers of certain items which we know to be satisfactory are listed in Appendix 5.

The question of cost is often difficult to resolve for several reasons. First, there is usually a wide range of equipment which will perform a given function. Although superior specifications may suggest a costly alternative, this may not be justified if only basic measurements are required. A rugged and simple instrument is often preferable to a complex one with higher capability. Secondly, the hidden costs involved in maintaining full working order should be estimated. Finally, the technical skill required to run the machine must be taken into account.

Before choosing any equipment, decisions have to be made regarding the type of tests to be performed, the measurements to be made, and the number of patients to be studied. In general it is best to start with simple techniques and to develop more complex facilities when experience has been gained.

ERGOMETERS

Cycles

Requirements for clinical use are as follows:
1. Constant and known power output at a given setting.
2. Adjustable height of handlebars, saddle, and the length of pedal stroke to accommodate patients of widely differing size.

3. Power output relatively independent of pedaling frequency.
4. A flywheel to maintain a cycling action in those patients unaccustomed to cycling.

TYPES AVAILABLE

A. *Mechanical.* In the simplest ergometers either one wheel of a modified bicycle is braked by a strap, or a flywheel is braked in a similar way (Fig. 5–1). The power output is calculated from the difference in tension between the two ends of the strap, the circumference of the wheel, and the pedaling rate. Cycle ergometers braked by a pad are virtually useless because accurate calibration is impossible.

In the most widely used machine both ends of the strap that brakes the flywheel are attached to a weighted physical balance (von Dobeln, 1954). This allows the tension to be adjusted simply and to be read off directly on a scale. Pedaling rate influences power output and should be controlled using a metronome. Friction in the bearings and other moving parts leads to a power output 8 to 10 per cent higher than calculated as above.

B. *Electromechanical.* In electrically braked and stabilized ergometers, work is performed against an electrically produced resistance. Specifications vary widely, and a flywheel may or may not be used. Usually, variations in pedaling frequency between 50 and 70 per minute do not affect the power output significantly. Calibration is more difficult than with mechanical ergometers, but it is extremely important where an accurately known and con-

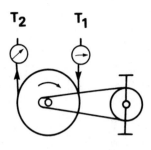

Figure 5–1 Calculation of power output — mechanically braked cycle ergometer.

$$W = (T_1 - T_2)\ \pi\ d\ f$$

where d = diameter of wheel
     f = frequency of rotation
  $T_1 - T_2$ = braking force

stant power output is required. Biological calibration (measurement of oxygen intake and heart rate in a subject whose performance has been established previously) is a method which can be used periodically. However, calibration is required at least once a year with a physical balance over the full range of work and pedaling frequencies. Suitable calibrating machines may be purchased or made in a laboratory workshop (Cumming and Alexander, 1968).

Our recommendation for clinical studies is an electromechanical ergometer, because precise regulation of pedaling rate is unnecessary. In addition, small increases in resistance may be made more accurately than with a mechanical ergometer. However, for field studies and epidemiological work, a mechanical ergometer is adequate and has the advantages of being portable, free from the need of an electrical supply, and less expensive.

Treadmills

REQUIREMENTS

1. Easily adjustable grade up to 25 per cent and speed up to 25 mph (40 km/hr) if high power outputs are to be studied. However, for most clinical purposes 14 per cent grade and 10 mph are sufficient (Fig. 5–2).
2. Accurate timing of speed.
3. Sturdy construction with handrails, side platforms, and a safety mechanism to stop the treadmill in an emergency.
4. Quiet operation.

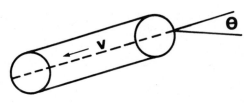

Figure 5–2 Calculation of power output—treadmill.

$$W = Wt \times v \times sine \ \theta$$

$$where \ v = speed$$

$$\theta = angle \ of \ elevation$$

There is a very wide range in the specifications and cost of tread-mills. The less powerful motors of cheaper machines are less reliable than those of more expensive machines, and it is therefore advisable to obtain a treadmill having higher specifications than those dictated by its laboratory usage. Most treadmills are bulky and require an electrical supply and are therefore not very suitable for field work.

Steps

REQUIREMENTS

1. One or two steps, adjustable in height between 2 to 12 inches.
2. Stable and covered with a nonslip surface.
3. Attached handrail.

A set of steps to these specifications is easily constructed. A convenient portable unit is described by Sharrock et al (1972).

MEASUREMENT OF VENTILATION

General Requirements

1. Accuracy over large ranges of volume and flow rates.
2. Low resistance and inertia.
3. Facility for electrical output suitable for a direct writing recorder.

Types of Equipment

ANEMOMETER

Anemometers (Wright, 1958) can be used for measurement of ventilation in simple exercise tests but are unreliable at high flow rates, when some gas may not be registered. In addition, they may be damaged by high flow rates and by water vapor and should be used on the inspired side of a respiratory valve. They are inconvenient to read, and an electrical output cannot be obtained.

DRY GAS METER

Models are available which have low resistance and sufficient accuracy at high flow rates. Some contain bellows, which tend to deteriorate, so they should be calibrated regularly. Although the volume registered by a full revolution is accurate, some nonlinearity may be present within a single revolution; these characteristics need to be studied for each meter. A potentiometer may be fitted to obtain an electrical output, or a photoelectric device may be used to correct for nonlinearity (Reynolds, 1968). They are best used for the measurement of inspired volume so that moist expired gas is not passed through them; also the washout volume is very large. The addition of a bellows between the subject and the meter improves the accuracy of measurement of total ventilation by damping the high flows through the meter (Cotes, 1965).

TISSOT SPIROMETER

Tissot Spirometers are of 50 to 600 liter capacity. Volume is recorded by measuring the vertical movement of the bell on a scale, from a kymograph, or from a potentiometer attached to one of the suspension pulleys. If expired gas is collected, the requisite flushing leads to unavoidable interruptions in the ventilation record, unless two spirometers are used.

PNEUMOTACHOGRAPH

Until recently, methods for integrating flow to obtain volume were insufficiently stable for accurate measurement during exercise, but it is now possible to adjust for electrical drift and to reset the signal if necessary after each breath. The output is affected by temperature changes and by the accumulation of water on the pneumotachograph screen. For these reasons this method is relatively unsuitable for routine exercise testing unless breath-by-breath measurements is required. The volume signal can be automatically processed with the output from gas analyzers to obtain breath-by-breath O_2 intake and CO_2 output (Wasserman et al, 1967). A suitable system has been detailed by Davies et al (1974).

We have found it helpful to have a system in which inspired ventilation is measured with a dry gas meter and expired gas is collected and measured in a Tissot spirometer. This allows continuous recording of inspired ventilation and intermittent recording of expired ventilation. An added advantage is that leaks in the respiratory valves are readily detected if both inspired and expired volumes are recorded.

MIXING AND COLLECTION OF EXPIRED
GAS FOR ANALYSIS

Ideally the system used to mix expired gas for continuous analysis and, if necessary, storage should:
1. mix gas rapidly and completely.
2. maintain constant composition of stored gas (that is, not leak and be impermeable to diffusion).
3. have a low resistance to flow.
4. accommodate at least 100 L but preferably 200 L.

Mixing Chambers of about 5 to 15 liter volume contain either a number of baffles (Fig. 5–3), or a fan for mixing expired gas. Their size is chosen with regard to the type of study to be performed: a large volume ensures good mixing but takes time to wash out; a small volume does not mix gases completely when the tidal volume is high. Expired gas composition is measured distal to the chamber and should not show tidal fluctuations.

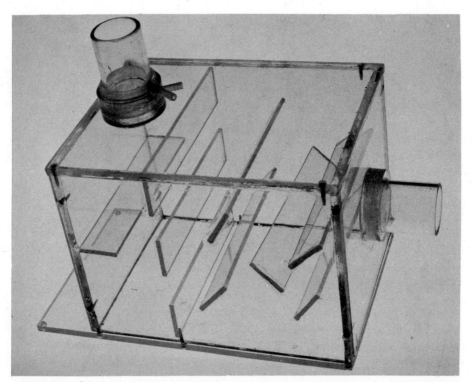

Figure 5–3   Mixing chamber for expired gas, size approximately 12 × 9 in, volume 5 liters.

Douglas Bags.   Bags of 50 to 200 liter capacity are suitable for the collection of expired gas. Polyvinyl and Mylar bags may be less permeable to CO_2 than the older canvas and rubber types, which usually deteriorate with time. Regular checks should be made to detect leakage and changes in gas concentration. Volume is measured after collection either by gas meter or Tissot spirometer.

Before a gas collection, bags should be evacuated by a vacuum pump or washed out by expired gas. They should be hung vertically to diminish resistance. If volume is to be measured, accuracy is increased by the use of a stop watch actuated by opening and closing the inlet tap (Åstrand and Rodahl, 1970). A bag-in-box system may be used to collect gas and record ventilation at the same time (Donald and Christie, 1949); it can be adapted inexpensively to provide multiple gas collections and automatic fill-empty cycles.

Tissot Spirometer.   Expired gas may be collected and stored for analysis, but because the spirometer has a large washout volume, repeated flushing with expired gas is necessary, and a fan is required for adequate mixing.

Although we recommend the Tissot spirometer because expired ventilation can be measured and gas mixed and stored for analysis, for reasons of cost or convenience, (in field studies, for example), Douglas bags may be preferable. Constantly changing expired gas composition, for example at the onset of exercise or where power output is changing frequently as in a Stage 1 test, is best monitored distal to a mixing chamber.

TUBING, VALVES, AND TAPS

The main requirement for the respiratory circuit, including gas meters and spirometers, is a low resistance. The total pressure due to resistance to inspiration or expiration should be less than 6 cm of H_2O with flows up to 300 L/min (that is, approximately 1 cm H_2O/L/sec).

Tubing

Tubing should be smooth internally and have an internal diameter of 3 to 5 cm so that its resistance is low. The total length of tubing used in a circuit should be as small as possible in order to minimize the total resistance, but angles, constructions, and junctions are more resistive than a straight length of tubing. It is better to permit longer tubing than to clutter the space around the subject. Tubing should be gas-sterilized periodically in order to prevent infection.

Valves

There is a wide selection of respiratory valves. The choice is dictated by a balance between dead-space volume and resistance. The smallest valves, for example the Ruben valve, generally have the highest resistance. Valves with very low resistance, such as the Otis-McKerrow valve (McKerrow and Otis, 1956), are required if maximal exercise is studied, but the dead-space volume is often high, variable, and not amenable to accurate measurement. A low dead space is required for accurate measurement of V_D/V_T ratio and also in children in whom a large dead space may compromise alveolar ventilation.

A plastic flap valve of the Lloyd type (Fig. 5–4) (Cunningham et al, 1965) achieves a good compromise between volume (46 ml) and resistance (less than 0.1 cm/L/sec) and is ideal for clinical testing.

Taps

Respiratory taps should be of similar bore to the valves and tubing, should prevent excessive turbulence due to angulation, and should be easy to operate. The most widely used taps are made of cast aluminum and have a 2 to 3 cm bore. Three-way taps having a 60° angle are preferable to those with a 90° angle. If the circuit is

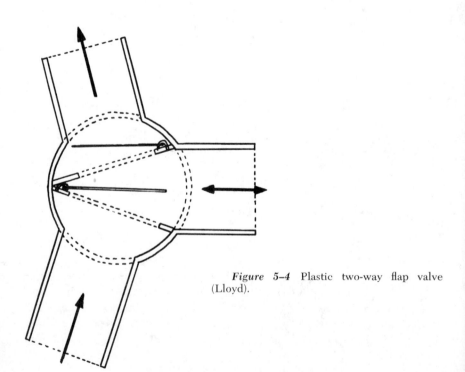

Figure 5–4 Plastic two-way flap valve (Lloyd).

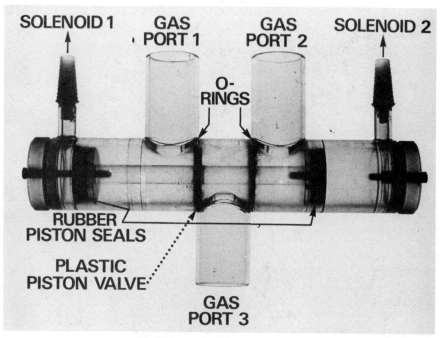

Figure 5–5   Solenoid-actuated pneumatic two-way tap.

to be controlled remotely, large-bore solenoid valves may be used. However, because they close forcibly, we use taps consisting of a piston moved by air pressure controlled remotely by small solenoids (Fig. 5–5). For rebreathing, a tap is placed between the mouthpiece and the respiratory valve; the volume of this assembly is kept low by using a sliding tap (Fig. 5–6) or a rotary four-channel tap (Lloyd and Wright, 1956). An alternative method to the pistons in the pneumatic taps described above is to use inflatable rubber balloons, which act in a similar way.

ANALYSIS OF MIXED EXPIRED GAS

If large numbers of exercise tests are being performed, physical gas analyzers permit more analyses to be carried out with a considerable saving of time. The basis of their accuracy, however, is dependent on accurate analysis of the calibrating gases, performed with a Lloyd-Haldane apparatus or the Scholander microanalyzer. There are many types of physical analyzers, and choice depends on several factors: the required response time; availability of service and repair facilities; the type of output required (meter, null point, analogue, or digital read-out); and cost.

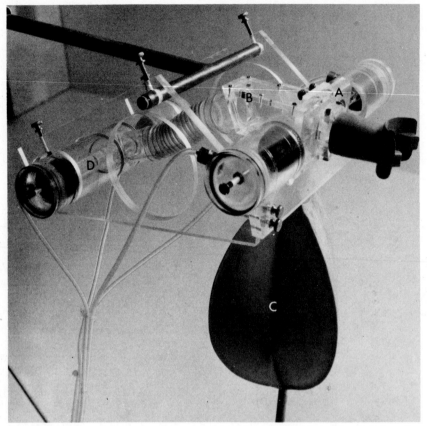

Figure 5-6 Respiratory valve and tap assembly showing (A) sliding tap for rebreathing, (B) two-way flap valve, (C) rebreathing bag, (D) two-way tap.

Carbon Dioxide

The measurement of carbon dioxide at the mouth during tidal breathing and during rebreathing requires a rapid analyzer. There are two main methods.

MASS SPECTROMETER

The mass spectrometer is expensive to install but has several advantages: extremely fast response, low sampling flow, linear output, and freedom from interference by other gases. Some difficulty may be experienced with water vapor, which travels through the sampling system at a lower rate than other gases. The mass spectrometer may also be used to measure a wide range of physiologically important gases. However, most laboratories will be unable to justify the cost, which is in excess of \$15,000 (£6000).

INFRARED CO$_2$ METER

Infrared CO$_2$ meters are less expensive, and the response time is a little slower but still fast enough to enable the rapid changes in gas concentration during breathing to be followed accurately. Since the infrared analyzer is not specific for carbon dioxide, some foreign gases such as nitrous oxide will interfere with its measurement. The oxygen concentration of the background gas has a small effect on the carbon dioxide concentration reading (Severinghaus, 1960), but this is overcome by calibrating with mixtures of carbon dioxide in concentrations of oxygen close to those in the gases to be analyzed. With careful calibration CO$_2$ can be analyzed with an accuracy of $\pm$ 0.05 per cent. Infrared meters with adequate specifications are obtainable from several manufacturers, and the only major difference between models lies in the linearity of the electrical output. Preferably the output should be linear to at least 12 per cent CO$_2$.

Oxygen

For most purposes in exercise testing there is no need for O$_2$ analysis to be rapid, but a high degree of accuracy is required. A *paramagnetic O$_2$ meter* is capable of analyzing O$_2$ with an accuracy of $\pm$ 0.03 per cent. Although the meter is not significantly affected by other respired gases, water vapor will dilute the sample. If dry calibration gases are used, the sample should be prepared by passing it over silica gel before analysis. Unless the analyzer has an electrical output it should use the null balance reading principle to provide the necessary accuracy.

There are several other methods for oxygen analysis, which, because of greater expense and instrument complexity, are best used only if rapid breath-by-breath analysis is required. These instruments include the rapid paramagnetic analyzer, the fuel cell oxygen analyzer, the polarographic electrode, and the mass spectrometer.

EQUIPMENT FOR MEASUREMENT OF MIXED VENOUS PCO$_2$ BY REBREATHING

A 5 liter anesthetic bag connected to the mouthpiece tap is filled with a known volume and concentration of carbon dioxide in oxygen

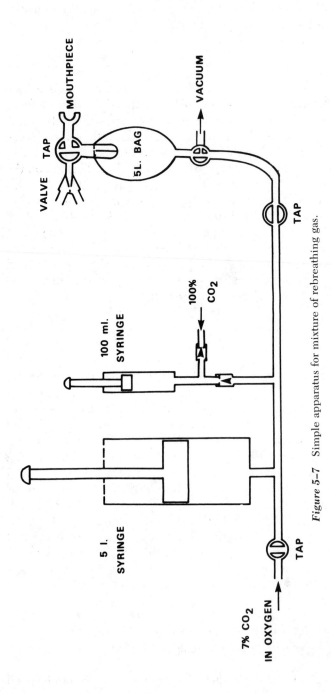

Figure 5-7 Simple apparatus for mixture of rebreathing gas.

obtained by using one of the methods listed below. The choice depends on the availability of engineering resources.

1. A series of mixtures of CO_2 in O_2 in 2 per cent steps between 7 and 15 per cent can be stored in gas cylinders and used to fill the rebreathing bag by opening the appropriate cylinder valve by hand. This method is convenient but expensive in the long run.
2. A system consisting of a 5 liter plastic piston attached to a cylinder of 7 per cent CO_2 in 93 per cent O_2 and a 100 ml plastic syringe attached to a cylinder of 100 per cent CO_2 enables any concentration of CO_2 in O_2 to be mixed in the required volume (Fig. 5–7). Although minor engineering may be required, this method is simple to use and cheap to run because commercially available CO_2 is used.
3. Gas pressure from cylinders of 7 per cent carbon dioxide in oxygen and 100 per cent carbon dioxide is regulated by high performance reducing valves. Solenoids controlled by time switches allow delivery of carbon dioxide in any concentration and volume to the rebreathing bag (Fig. 5–8). Although more engineering is needed with this method of preparing the gas mixture for rebreathing, it is recommended because of its speed and ease of operation.

BLOOD GAS ANALYSIS

Several electrode systems for the measurement of blood gases and pH are capable of accurate analysis of small samples of blood (Severinghaus, 1962). We will not attempt to review these systems, which all use the same analytical principles. In general it is best to obtain a simple system which is easy to maintain. The accuracy of analysis is established by tonometry; PCO_2 and PO_2 in the physiological range should be analyzed with an accuracy of ± 1.5 mm Hg. Some O_2 electrodes will be found to read PO_2 in blood a few mm Hg lower than in gas, and a correction is applied for this gas-blood difference, once it has been established by tonometry.

Several methods exist for measurement of blood O_2 saturation. In general if PO_2 and pH are measured, O_2 saturation may be calculated with reasonable accuracy (± 2 per cent). More accurate measurement is seldom required except for specific research reasons. The indirect method of ear oximetry may be useful in routine testing if completely bloodless methods are required. We recommend individual calibration for any given subject using a rebreathing method (Lal et al, 1966).

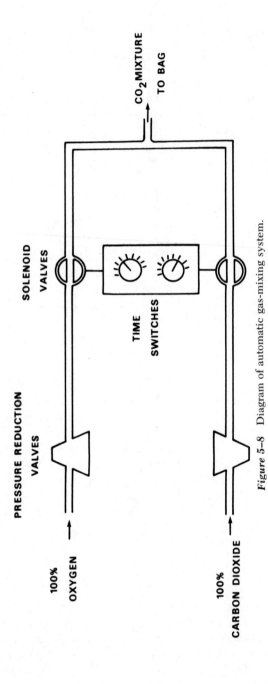

Figure 5–8 Diagram of automatic gas-mixing system.

BLOOD PRESSURE

Although the measurement of systemic arterial pressure by auscultation or palpation is subject to error, for most purposes changes in systolic pressure with exercise can be measured with sufficient accuracy by trained observers. Measurement of diastolic pressure by this method often is unreliable.

If arterial blood is being sampled with an indwelling catheter, arterial pressure may be measured using a pressure transducer and recorder.

Measurement of pulmonary arterial pressure through a thin catheter requires a pressure transducer and accurate calibration; this is a well established technique which should not be difficult to use in any laboratory in which vascular catheterization is regularly performed.

ELECTROCARDIOGRAPHY

The electrocardiograph is preferred for the measurement of cardiac frequency over the less accurate measurement obtained by palpation of the radial or carotid pulse. Rate is measured from a recorder output or may be displayed automatically in digital form. Display of the electrocardiograph is essential in monitoring rhythm and in recognizing changes in the ST segment and T wave: high quality recordings, free from drift and interference, are necessary for diagnostic use. These are obtained by reducing skin resistance with abrasion, by using correctly placed electrodes which minimize artifact, and through appropriate signal conditioning.

Although the record obtained from an electrode in the V_5 position with an indifferent electrode on the manubrium sternum or forehead identifies 90 per cent of all ischemic electrocardiographic responses (McHenry et al, 1972), occasionally additional information is obtained from other leads. A laboratory used extensively for testing coronary patients requires facilities for recording of Frank X, Y, and Z leads. Although muscle artifact may be a problem, the addition of a recording from the inferior aspect of the heart is an advantage; similar information is obtained as in a 12-lead recording.

A variety of electrodes is available. Best results are obtained from electrodes attached to the skin by circular adhesive pads that leave a gap between the electrode and the skin, which is filled by conducting jelly. Alternatives range from disposable stainless steel mesh electrodes to silver-silver chloride electrodes, which in our experience are very satisfactory. The quality of electrocardiograph recordings is influenced by several types of "noise," which need to be reduced to a minimum if recordings are to be interpreted reliably. Cyclic noise at a frequency of 60 cps may be reduced by band pass filters chosen for their ability to attenuate noise without distorting the complexes. Random noise and baseline shift are more difficult to deal with, although they are reduced by good skin preparation; in these types of noise digital computer smoothing has been found to be a powerful tool. The computer also may be programed to make measurements of ST depression and its duration (Rautaharju, 1969).

RECORDERS

A recorder is used to collect basic data using the electrical output from the electrocardiograph, O_2 and CO_2 analyzers, and a gas meter or spirometer.

Desirable characteristics of a recorder are as follows:

1. At least four, and preferably six channels.
2. Direct writing so that data are available immediately.
3. Rectilinear writing system.
4. Flat frequency response to 50 Hz.
5. Resolution greater than 1 per cent of the full scale deflection.
6. Zero suppression.

If a large volume of studies is contemplated the cost of recorder paper may be important, as there is a wide variation among brands. Many recorders meet most of the preceding specifications, and a few meet all. The requirements which may not be immediately obvious are those related to the measurement of CO_2. The reading accuracy for this should be at least 1 mm of pen deflection for 1 mm Hg PCO_2: as the highest levels of PCO_2 approach 100 mm Hg during rebreathing, a full-scale deflection of at least 10 cm is required. In order to obtain this, more than one channel of the recorder may be required with zero suppression in one channel.

RESUSCITATION EQUIPMENT

The laboratory should be equipped to meet an emergency, and personnel should be capable of maintaining life until the patient can be managed by a cardiac team. The following is a list of the equipment required.

1. Drugs for intravenous use: adrenaline, atropine, aminophylline, digoxin, isoprenaline, xylocaine, propranolol, hydrocortisone, procaine amide, sodium bicarbonate, calcium gluconate.
2. Syringes, intravenous infusion sets, and glucose saline.
3. Hand ventilator, such as the Ambu bag.
4. Airways, endotracheal tubes, laryngoscope.
5. Rapid (less than 2 min) access to D.C. defibrillator.
6. Oxygen.

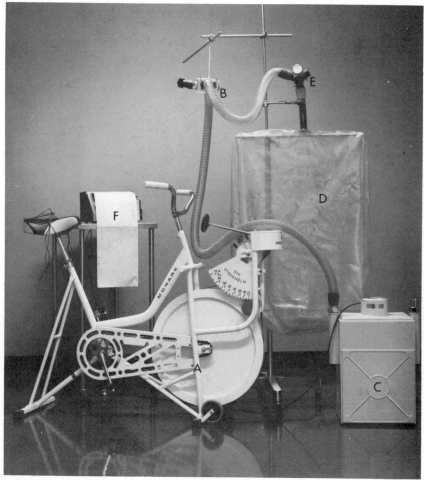

Figure 5-9 Simple system suitable for exercise testing. (A) mechanically braked cycle ergometer, (B) Otis-McKerrow valve, (C) dry gas meter measuring inspired volume and fitted with potentiometer, (D) Douglas bag collecting expired gas, (E) stopwatch for accurate timing of expired gas collections, (F) recorder for electrocardiograph and potentiometer signals.

SUMMARY

The requirements for a laboratory offering a clinical exercise testing service follow from the recommendations above. Exact cost has not been detailed due to variations in equipment, manufacturers, and location. The following is a summary of equipment needed and approximate cost of systems capable of performing the staged procedures outlined in this chapter.

Stage 1. An electromechanical cycle ergometer; dry gas meter; low resistance valve, taps and tubing; electrocardiograph signal conditioning; three-channel recorder; resuscitation equipment. Cost: (U.S.) $8000 to $10,000 (£3000 to £4000) (Fig. 5–9).

Stage 2. Additional equipment—infrared CO_2 analyzer; paramagnetic O_2 analyzer; Tissot spirometer; three extra recording channels. Cost of total system: (U.S.) $20,000 to $25,000 (£8,000 to £10,000) (Figs. 5–10 and 5–11).

Stage 3. Additional equipment—blood gas electrodes; spectrophotometer for lactate determination. Cost of total system: (U.S.) $25,000 to $35,000 (£10,000 to £14,000).

Addition of on-line analytical and computational equipment

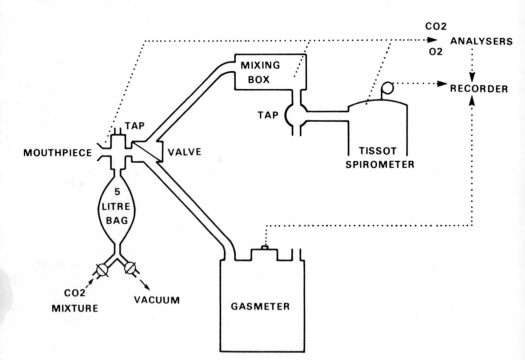

Figure 5–10   Diagram of equipment required for Stage 2 exercise tests.

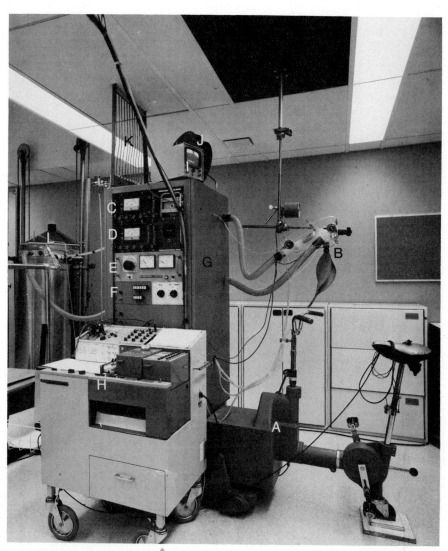

Figure 5–11 System for Stages 2 and 3 exercise tests. (A) electrically braked ergometer, (B) mouthpiece assembly with rebreathing bag on adjustable rig, (C) CO_2 analyzer, (D) O_2 analyzer, (E) ergometer control, (F) solenoid controls, (G) cabinet containing analyzers, dry gas meter, mixing chamber (not seen), and control panels, (H) recorder, (I) oscilloscope, (J) fan (K) calibration gas inlets, (L) tissot spirometer.

described in Chapter 7 would increase costs of any of these systems by (U.S.) $10,000 to $20,000 (£4000 to £8000).

The laboratory should be at least 300 square feet in area, not including analytical laboratory space, and it should be possible to control temperature to within a range of 19 to 23° C.

Equipment should be arranged bearing two main aims in mind. First, the subject should be freely accessible from all sides, and recording equipment should be largely out of sight. Secondly, the operator should have easy access to all controls and recording equipment and be able to keep the subject in full view without moving. Equipment which does not require manipulation during the test such as gas meters, spirometers, gas tanks, and computer should be remote from the area.

References

Åstrand, P.-O., and Rodahl, K.: Textbook of Work Physiology. New York, McGraw-Hill Book Co., 1970.

Cotes, J. E.: Lung Function. (Blackwell Scientific Pubns.) Philadelphia, F. A. Davis Co., 1965.

Cumming, G. R., and Alexander, W. D.: The calibration of bicycle ergometers. Can. J. Physiol. Pharm. 46:917–919, 1968.

Cunningham, D. J. C., Elliott, D. H., Lloyd, B. B., Miller, J. P. and Young, J. M.: A comparison of the effects of oscillating and steady alveolar partial pressures of oxygen and carbon dioxide on the pulmonary ventilation. J. Physiol. 179:498–508, 1965.

Davies, E. E., Hahn, H. L., Spiro, S. G. and Edwards, R. H. T.: A new technique for recording respiratory transients at the start of exercise. Resp. Physiol. 20:69–79, 1974.

Dobeln, W. von: A simple bicycle ergometer. J. Appl. Physiol. 7:222–224, 1954.

Donald, K. W., and Christie, R. V.: A new method of clinical spirometry. Clin. Sci. 8:21, 1949.

Lal, S., Gebbie, T. and Campbell, E. J. M.: Simple methods for improving the value of oximetry in the study of pulmonary oxygen uptake. Thorax 21:50–56, 1966.

Lloyd, B. B., and Wright, T. A.: A four channel tap for use in human respiratory studies. J. Physiol. (London) 133:34, 1956.

McHenry, P. L., Phillips, J. F. and Knoebel, S. B.: Correlation of computer-quantitated treadmill exercise electrocardiogram with arteriographic location of coronary artery disease. Am. J. Cardiol. 30:747–752, 1972.

McKerrow, C. B., and Otis, A. B.: Low resistance value for hyperventilation. J. Appl. Physiol. 9:497, 1956.

Rautaharju, P. M., Friedrich, H. and Wolf, H.: Measurement and interpretation of exercise electrocardiograms. In Shephard, R. J. (ed.): Frontiers of Fitness. Springfield, Ill., Charles C Thomas, Publisher, 1971.

Reynolds, J. A.: A method of recording pulmonary ventilation. J. Sci. Instrum. 1:433–450, 1968.

Severinghaus, J. W.: Methods of measurement of blood and gas carbon dioxide during anaesthesia. Anaesthesiology 21:717–726, 1960.

Severinghaus, J. W.: Electrodes for blood and gas PCO_2, PO_2 and blood pH. Acta Anaesth. Scand. 11:208–219, 1962.

Sharrock, N., Garrett, H. L., and Mann, G. V.: Practical exercise test for physical fitness and cardiac performance. Am. J. Cardiol. 30:727–732, 1972.

Wasserman, K., Van Kessel, A. L. and Burton, G.: Interaction of physiological mechanisms during exercise. J. Appl. Physiol. 22:71–85, 1967.

Wright, B. M.: A respiratory anemometer. J. Physiol. (London) 127:25, 1958.

Chapter Six

PERFORMANCE OF EXERCISE TESTS

The present chapter describes the general conduct of exercise tests and details the procedures outlined in Chapter 3.

SAFETY PRECAUTIONS

The risks to the patient of an exercise test are very small, provided that some simple precautions are observed. Although the danger of myocardial infarction or serious arrhythmia is estimated at about 1 in 10,000 submaximal tests (Rochmis and Blackburn, 1971), the incidence increases with maximal tests and rises to about 1 in 2500 in patients who have suffered from a myocardial infarct in the past (Shephard, 1970).

Although the referring physician takes some responsibility for deciding that an exercise test does not carry undue risk, often he will be unfamiliar with the procedure. Thus a physician experienced in the procedure should always supervise the test and should review the patient's history and physical findings. It may be helpful to obtain more information from the referring doctor before proceeding with the test. Some patients may have symptoms which so severely limit exercise that testing may produce very little useful information and be too distressing for the patient. In such cases it may be necessary to abandon or defer the test. Myocardial infarction within the previous three months, cardiomyopathy, severe aortic stenosis, and uncontrolled cardiac failure or arrhythmias are generally regarded as situations in which the risks may outweigh the value of the test in the clinical management of the patient. In any patient over 40 years of age suspected of heart disease, a 12-lead electrocardiograph should precede the test to exclude recent ischemic changes and to provide a base line should any ill effect follow the test.

Indications to Stop an Exercise Test

1. SYMPTOMS AND GENERAL SIGNS
    A. Increasing chest pain suggestive of angina.
    B. Severe dyspnea.
    C. Extreme fatigue.
    D. Dizziness or faintness.
    E. Marked apprehension, mental confusion, or lack of coordination.
    F. Sudden onset of pallor and sweating, or of cyanosis.
2. ELECTROCARDIOGRAPHIC SIGNS
    A. Frequent ventricular premature beats, particularly where they occur in the T wave; ventricular paroxysmal tachycardia; paroxysmal atrial tachycardia; atrial fibrillation when absent at rest.
    B. Second or third degree heart block.
    C. Symmetrical T wave inversion of 0.3 mv or more not present at rest; ST segment depressions of 0.2 mv or more with horizontal or downward slope of ST segment; or horizontal ST segment elevations of 0.2 mv or more (see p. 108).
3. BLOOD PRESSURE
    A. Fall of more than 25 mm Hg in systolic pressure.
    B. Systolic blood pressure in excess of 280 mm Hg.

The observers should always be alert to the possibility of the untoward effects of the procedure, and the laboratory must have facilities for resuscitation as outlined on page 78. During the test the patient and the electrocardiogram are observed continuously, and the test is terminated if these untoward symptoms or signs develop. If the patient is known or suspected to have heart disease, a predetermined heart rate is not exceeded unless the doctor supervising the test considers it safe to do so. It has been agreed that this limit should be 85 per cent of the maximum heart rate, predicted from the patient's age (p. 35), in patients with ischemic heart disease (American Heart Association, 1972).

After completion of the test, the electrocardiogram is observed for at least five minutes for post-exercise changes in the electrocardiograph. If any complications occur, the subject remains in the laboratory until they have cleared. On rare occasions it may be wise to admit the patient to hospital for further observation and management; in our experience this was required once, for a patient with aortic valve disease who developed early signs of pulmonary edema. It must be emphasized that it is in the best interests of the patient and the laboratory to establish a careful routine to prevent complications insofar as possible, to detect them promptly, and to deal with them adequately. This is not because the true risks are high but because patients referred for exercise tests inevitably include a number who are liable to coincidental deterioration. The charge of *post hoc ergo propter hoc* is easier to refute if a laboratory discipline has been established.

CONDUCTING THE TESTS

We have already explained our preference for the cycle ergometer. The details which follow apply to tests in which this instrument is used, but similar principles pertain to the use of treadmills or steps. The graph in Appendix 3 provides data for interconversion of load settings.

Preliminary Procedures

Time allowed for checking and setting up equipment before the patient arrives ensures that the procedure runs smoothly. Some time should be devoted to explaining the test and describing the equipment to the patient to reduce possible anxiety. We find it helpful to enclose a short letter with the appointment notice, explaining what will be done, suggesting suitable clothing, and asking the patient to refrain from taking exercise or eating a meal during the two hours preceding the test.

Measurements are made to help predict the expected response in the subject, assuming he represents the normal population. To the standard data of age, sex, height, and weight should be added spirometry (vital capacity and FEV_1) so that the maximal voluntary ventilation can be estimated; skin-fold thicknesses; and thigh circumference, to estimate lean body mass (Cotes et al, 1969). Blood hemoglobin level should also be known, because it is used in the calculation of cardiac output and is one of the variables which may influence oxygen transport. Other techniques may be helpful in some situations but are more complex and rarely needed for an adequate assessment of patients. These include radiographic heart volume (Reindell, 1966), which yields an index of cardiac stroke volume; total hemoglobin by the carbon monoxide technique (Sjöstrand, 1948), reflecting the circulating blood volume; and measurement of total body potassium using a total body counter for K40 (Wolmersley et al, 1972), the most accurate index of muscle mass. A consent form is signed by the patient if arterial blood is to be sampled.

Test Procedure

Electrocardiographic electrodes are usually placed on the left chest in the lead V_S position and on the forehead or thoracic spine. Where X, Y, and Z leads are to be recorded, electrodes are placed in the midaxillary line on both sides, on the lower sternum, over the lower thoracic spine, and on the forehead. Excessive chest hair may need to be shaved, and the skin under the electrode should be abraded with a nylon scourer. If there is much subcutaneous fat, an elastic net, or, in women, a well-fitting brassiere, will help to prevent electrode movement. The electrocardiograph record is standardized in the usual manner (1 mv = 1 cm deflection).

The patient sits on the ergometer, and the position of the saddle and mouthpiece are adjusted for comfort. The saddle height should be such that the knee is almost fully extended at the bottom of the pedal stroke. Small saddles are used for children and if possible the pedal stroke is reduced appropriately. The mouthpiece and respiratory valve assembly are positioned so that the patient is leaning slightly forward but so that the neck is not uncomfortably extended. Attention to these details will gain the patient's confidence and cooperation.

STAGE 1 — PROGRESSIVE POWER OUTPUT TEST

A suitable initial power output is 100 kpm/min (about 16 watts), which can be used for each increment in most adult patients and in children over 150 cm in height; this should be halved in sick patients and in children of less than 120 cm in height (Godfrey et al, 1971). As a general rule the initial and incremental power output should approximate 10 per cent of the subject's predicted maximum. Most electrically braked ergometers indicate the pedaling rate, which should be kept at 50 to 60 revolutions per minute. Occasionally, where difficulty is experienced in keeping a constant rate, it is helpful to have the patient pedal in time to a metronome or to spoken instruction. With a treadmill an equivalent progression of power outputs should be chosen — a useful protocol is that described by Bruce (1971).

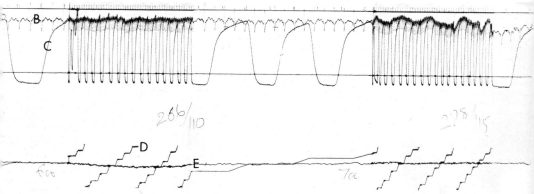

Figure 6–1 Two-minute segment from recording obtained in Stage 1 test, showing data obtained at 600 and 700 kpm/min.

A, timer (seconds); B, electrocardiograph; C, CO_2 in gas sampled from the mouthpiece of valve assembly; D, dry gas meter (inspired ventilation); E, O_2 in gas sampled from mixing chamber.

Blood pressure is noted by observer. Note that paper speed is increased for last 10 seconds of each minute.

The patient is observed during the initial period of the test and encouraged to breathe slowly if obvious hyperventilation is noticed. During the last 15 seconds of each minute, a record is obtained of ventilation and heart rate; the electrocardiograph is inspected for an abnormal electrical pattern, by increasing the recorder paper speed to obtain a clear tracing; and, if analyzers for CO_2 and O_2 are used (see below), the mixed expired gas concentrations are recorded. The type of record obtained is shown in Figure 6–1. The power output is increased at the end of each minute, and the test is continued until the patient stops because of symptoms, or the observer ends the procedure according to the guidelines described earlier. Throughout the test the patient is encouraged to pedal steadily and regularly, is kept informed regarding progress in the test, and is constantly reassured regarding the performance of his heart and lungs. There is no doubt that communication of this sort increases confidence and helps patients to perform to the best of their ability, although there is no point in trying to coax patients past the stage at which they are distressed.

STAGE 2—CONSTANT POWER OUTPUT TEST WITHOUT BLOOD SAMPLING

In order to assess the evolution of the response to exercise, at least two work rates should be studied. If information is available from a Stage 1 procedure, levels of 1/3 and 2/3 of the highest work rate reached in that test are chosen, which usually means an initial power output of 100 to 400 kpm/min with increases of similar amounts, although smaller values may be needed for children or severely disabled adults. The preparation is similar to the progressive test and the routine is as follows (Fig. 6–2). The O_2 and CO_2 analyzers are calibrated. Two channels of the recorder are used for CO_2: on one the gain is adjusted so that a full scale deflection is obtained for 0 to 7 per cent CO_2; on the other, zero is suppressed to read CO_2 between 6 and 12 per cent CO_2. Three gases are used for each channel in order to construct calibration curves (Fig. 6–2A). The full scale deflection for ventilation signals is adjusted for a volume of 10 liters. When the patient is accustomed to breathing through the mouthpiece and is comfortable, heart rate and mixed venous P_{CO_2} are measured (Fig. 6–2B). Little information is obtained from the measurement of resting ventilation, O_2 uptake, and CO_2 output, and these are best omitted owing to the length of time most patients take to settle into a steady state at rest. The patient starts to exercise, and the heart rate is measured every half-minute (Fig. 6–2C). A variation of less than ± 5 beats during a period of one minute is sufficient indication of a steady state. Oxygen and carbon dioxide concentrations in expired gas are monitored by analyzing gas distal to a mixing chamber or from a Tissot spirometer. A variation in expired CO_2 and O_2 of less than ± 0.1 per cent absolute concentration indicates a steady state of CO_2 output and O_2 intake (Fig. 6–2D).

During this time expired gas is passed through the Tissot spirometer to wash out the dead space. If a Douglas bag is used it is evacuated using a source of negative pressure. The exact length of time for collection is measured, and taps are closed during the inspiratory phase of breathing. When heart rate and expired gas composition have been steady for one minute, expired gas is collected in the Tissot spirometer or Douglas bag for a period of one minute, during which time end tidal P_{CO_2} is recorded (Fig. 6–2E). The rebreathing bag is prepared with a suitable mixture of CO_2 in O_2 towards the end of the collection period, and rebreathing is performed when the expired gas collection has been completed (Fig. 6–2F). A tap between the valve assembly and spirometer or bag is closed to prevent mixture of the rebreathed gas with the expired gas collection. As outlined below, an acceptable estimate of mixed venous P_{CO_2} can be obtained with one or two rebreathes. When a suitable equilibration has been obtained, the contents of the Tissot spirometer or Douglas bag are analyzed for CO_2 and O_2, and the analyzers are calibrated. The patient is then asked to indicate a subjective assessment of the work as outlined below.

Unless there is a contraindication such as the presence of ischemic heart disease, in which case it is wise to separate work periods by short periods of rest or loadless pedaling, the work rate is increased and the routine repeated.

STAGE II TEST ROUTINE

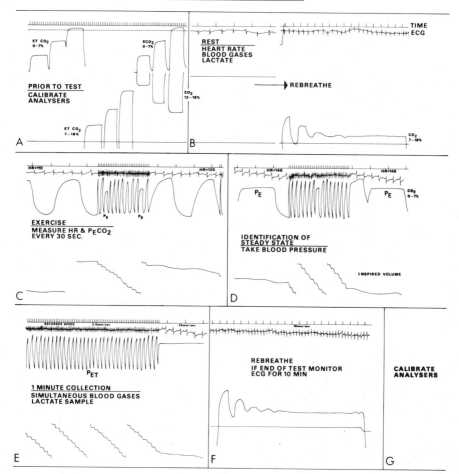

Figure 6-2   Examples of recordings made during an exercise test (⅓ actual size).

At the end of the test the gas analyzers are recalibrated. If gas from the Tissot spirometer, the mixing chamber, and the mouthpiece are sampled through separate tubing, separate calibrations should be made through each of them. Variations in the length of sample lines and the amount of condensed water vapor contained in them may lead to differences in analyzer output.

Although this description has been written with cycle ergometer tests in mind, the principles and methods are easily applicable to treadmill testing.

STAGE 3—CONSTANT POWER OUTPUT TEST WITH BLOOD SAMPLING

As outlined in Chapter 3, blood sampling increases the amount of information obtained from an exercise test. Several methods are available and are described below.

In contrast to the bloodless Stage 2 study, the additional information obtained from blood analysis make a resting study worthwhile, as the change with exercise in V_D/V_T ratio and A-a Po_2 difference may then be examined.

After the patient is breathing comfortably at rest, mixed expired gas is monitored until a steady state of expired gas composition is achieved. Expired gas and arterial blood are collected during a three-minute period in order to minimize the effect of variations in ventilation, which occur in many patients during the resting state. At the end of collection, rebreathing Pco_2 is measured, and exercise is started. The Stage 2 test routine is followed, and arterial blood is sampled at the same time that a collection of expired gas is made under steady state conditions (Fig. 6–2E).

STAGE 4—CONSTANT POWER OUTPUT TEST WITH PULMONARY FLOAT CATHETER

A similar procedure to the Stage 3 test is followed, with recording of pulmonary artery pressure during the steady state. Close attention should be paid to the electrocardiograph for cardiac arrhythmias, and if runs of ventricular premature beats occur, the catheter should be withdrawn.

Measurements and Calculations

Calculations are detailed in the Appendix and are outlined here to give an appreciation of the principles involved (Fig. 6–3).

A recorder output (Fig. 6–2) is obtained for the following channels of basic information:

1. Time in seconds.
2. Electrocardiograph.
3. Inspired air volume.
4. Expired gas volume (Tissot spirometer, except where expired gas is collected in Douglas bags).
5. Carbon dioxide—deflections for calibration gases, mixed expired gas, end tidal gas, and CO_2 during the rebreathing procedure.
6. O_2 concentration in mixed expired gas may be recorded in a

similar manner to CO_2, or the concentration may be read directly from the O_2 analyzer.

Using these deflections the following data are calculated:

1. Cardiac frequency (f_c)—from the electrocardiograph.
2. Ventilation ($\dot{V}_E$)—from the volume records, making appropriate corrections so that the measurement made at ambient temperature (ATPS) is converted to the conventional value expressed at body temperature (BTPS). Tidal volume (V_T) is then derived by simple division, using the frequency of breathing.
3. CO_2 concentration in mixed expired and end tidal gas and during the rebreathing equilibrium from the CO_2 deflections and the calibrating gas concentrations.
4. Carbon dioxide output ($\dot{V}CO_2$) from the expired CO_2 concentration and the expired ventilation, on this occasion expressed at standard temperature (0° C) and pressure (760 mm Hg) (STPD).
5. Oxygen intake ($\dot{V}O_2$) from the difference between the amount of O_2 inspired (inspired ventilation × inspired O_2 concentration) and the amount expired (expired ventilation × expired O_2 concentration). Although inspired and expired ventilation may be measured separately, use is usually made of the fact that for practical purposes the amount of nitrogen inspired equals that expired. This allows inspired ventilation to be calculated from measurements of expired ventilation and vice-versa.
6. The respiratory exchange ratio (R) by dividing CO_2 output by O_2 intake.
7. Mixed venous PCO_2 ($P_{\bar{v}}CO_2$) from the equilibrium PCO_2 during rebreathing.
8. The increase in blood lactate concentration is estimated by calculating the CO_2 output in excess of that produced from aerobic metabolism, by allowing for changes in the body CO_2 stores as reflected in changes in mixed venous PCO_2 (Chap. 11).

When arterial or capillary blood is sampled (Stage 3 procedure), the following additional measurements are made:

1. Arterial PCO_2 (P_aCO_2).
2. Arterial PO_2 (P_aO_2).
3. Arterial pH.
4. Arterial lactate concentration.

From these the following additional variables are calculated:

1. Alveolar ventilation from $\dot{V}CO_2$ and P_aCO_2.
2. V_D/V_T ratio from P_aCO_2 and P_ECO_2.

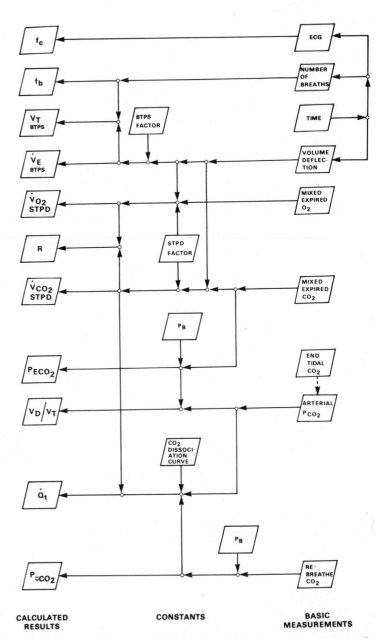

Figure 6–3 Scheme to illustrate derivation of results from the basic measurements made in an exercise test.

3. Cardiac output from $\dot{V}CO_2$, $P_{\bar{v}}CO_2$, and P_aCO_2.
4. Alveolar PO_2 (P_AO_2) from P_aCO_2 and R.
5. Alveolar-arterial PO_2 difference (A-a PO_2).
6. $\dot{Q}_{va}/\dot{Q}_t$ from $\dot{V}O_2$, $\dot{Q}_t$, P_AO_2, and P_aO_2.
7. Arterial O_2 saturation from PO_2 and pH, using the O_2 dissociation curve (Kelman and Nunn, 1968).
8. Arterial bicarbonate concentration from P_aCO_2 and pH.

Although this list of information obtained in studies where blood is sampled is impressive, knowledge of PCO_2 in mixed expired and mixed venous blood, both obtained without blood sampling in the Stage 2 procedure, will allow the limits to be placed on arterial PCO_2. From this the range of possible values for the derived variables can be defined and often will be narrow enough for conclusions to be drawn regarding their normality. The use of bloodless measurements is detailed in Chapter 10, with examples to illustrate the approach. When arterial blood is not sampled, in Stage 2 studies, an estimate may be obtained of P_aCO_2 from $P_{ET}CO_2$ in subjects free of lung dysfunction, or by assuming a normal value for the V_D/V_T ratio.

SPECIAL PROCEDURES

Most of the techniques involved in the procedures described above are simple and well known, and accurate results will be obtained if basic rules are followed to ensure that analysis, data reduction, and calculations are properly performed. Accuracy in gas analysis of expired air and blood is crucial to the Stage 2 and 3 procedures, and some checks to ensure this are listed (p. 103). Of the measurements discussed, the rebreathing method for mixed venous PCO_2 may be unfamiliar, but it has been described in principle in Chapter 4.

Procedure for Estimating Mixed Venous PCO_2

The procedure is explained to the subject before exercise is begun, and a rebreathe is performed at rest to accustom the patient to the transient sensation of dyspnea which may occur. The patient is reassured that oxygen is present in the bag and that rebreathing will last a few seconds only. Rebreathes are performed from a 5 liter anesthetic bag attached to a tap between mouth and breathing valve (Fig. 5–6) and containing a mixture of CO_2 in O_2 at a volume equivalent to about 1.5 times the subject's tidal volume.

TABLE 6-1 SUGGESTED INITIAL BAG CO_2 CONCENTRATIONS REQUIRED TO OBTAIN REBREATHING CO_2 EQUILIBRIUM

POWER OUTPUT		O_2 UPTAKE LITERS/MIN	END-TIDAL PCO_2 MM HG	BAG CO_2 CONCENTRATION %
KPM/MIN	WATTS			
300	50	1	40	11.5
			30	10.5
600	100	1.5	40	12
			30	11
900	150	2.2	40	13
			30	12
1200	200	3.0	40	14
			30	13

The concentration of CO_2 in the bag which is required to obtain equilibration with mixed venous PCO_2 may be chosen from the data given in Table 6–1, which applies to normal subjects. In cases where the mixed venous PCO_2 is suspected of being higher than normal, because of low cardiac output or hypoventilation, these concentrations should be increased by 1 to 2 per cent. The mixture can be prepared in various ways (see Chap. 5).

The tap at the mouthpiece is switched at the end of an expiration so that the patient inspires from the bag. If the breathing rate is slow (less than 30/min), the patient is asked to breathe more rapidly in order to facilitate mixing of gases between the bag and the lung, but complete emptying of the bag should be avoided, owing to the effect of negative pressure on the CO_2 analyzer (Fig. 6–4). This effect may

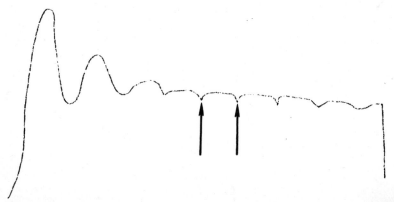

Figure 6–4   The effect of negative pressure on the CO_2 analyzer, due to emptying of the bag or to collapse at the neck of the bag.

also be caused by collapse at the neck of the bag, which is remedied with a wire cage.

Rebreathing is continued for 20 seconds at rest or 15 seconds on exercise. Gas is sampled continuously from the mouthpiece, and the record obtained from the CO_2 analyzer is examined for an equilibrium (see opposite). The bag is then emptied either manually or by connecting it to a vacuum source. If necessary, another mixture is prepared which has a different bag volume or CO_2 concentration chosen from the pattern obtained as outlined below.

INTERPRETATION OF THE RECORD

Various patterns may be obtained during rebreathing (Fig. 6–5) (Jones et al, 1967).

1. The P_{CO_2} rises continuously and sharply owing to continuous evolution of carbon dioxide from the mixed venous blood, showing that the initial concentration of carbon dioxide in the bag was too low to obtain an equilibrium.

2. A transient equilibrium lasting for one complete breathing cycle only is followed by a rise in P_{CO_2} before recirculation of blood is expected. This pattern indicates a transient equilibrium between the rebreathing bag and the alveolar gas but not with mixed venous blood. Because the P_{CO_2} is less than the blood P_{CO_2}, CO_2 is added to the system from mixed venous blood before recirculation. Recirculation will not appreciably affect the mixed venous P_{CO_2} before 10 seconds of rebreathing during exercise (Sowton et al, 1968).

3. A sustained constant P_{CO_2} is obtained that lasts until at least 10 seconds after the start of rebreathing. This record indicates an equilibrium between the P_{CO_2} in the bag, alveolar gas, and mixed venous blood.

4. The initial bag P_{CO_2} may be so high that an equilibrium is not obtained before recirculation. Knowledge of the recirculation time dictates that equilibrium should be obtained within three breaths (or six seconds) and maintained until 15 seconds after the start of rebreathing at rest, or 10 seconds during exercise.

If a true equilibrium is not obtained, rebreathing is repeated, using a CO_2 mixture dictated by the pattern obtained; if the initial mixture was too low (Patterns 1 or 2), a higher concentration of CO_2 is used in the second mixture. If the CO_2 concentration in the bag for the first rebreathe was too high (Pattern 4), the bag for the next rebreathe should contain a lower concentration. Unless the pattern indicates that the initial CO_2 concentration was highly inappropriate, the CO_2 concentration of the bag is increased or reduced by 2 per cent CO_2. At least 30 seconds is allowed between successive maneuvers to avoid the transient elevation of mixed venous P_{CO_2}.

Selecting the mixtures by this method usually allows an equi-

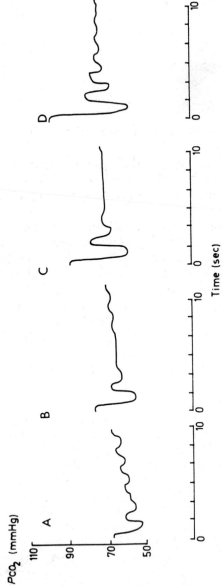

Figure 6-5 Records of P_{CO_2} during the rebreathing of four mixtures of increasing CO_2 concentration to show the equilibration patterns that may occur.

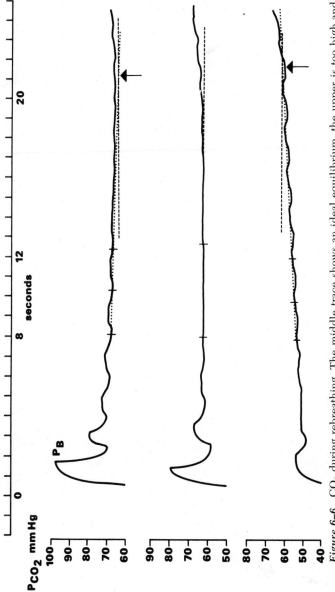

Figure 6–6 CO_2 during rebreathing. The middle trace shows an ideal equilibrium, the upper is too high and lower is too low. Extrapolation of the lines joining the end-expiratory values between 8 and 12 secs of rebreathing intersect at the same point, at 20–22 secs (indicated by arrows) in each example.

librium to be achieved with one or two rebreathes. If an ideal equilibration has not been obtained even though two rebreathes have been performed using initial CO_2 concentrations, one of which was too high and the other too low, the equilibrium value may be obtained by joining the end tidal PCO_2 values between 8 and 12 seconds of rebreathing and extrapolating to the point of intersection. This value will be within ± 2 mm of the true equilibrium value (Fig. 6–6) (Jones and Rebuck, 1973). Because this intersection is found to occur between 20 and 25 seconds of rebreathing, a further method of estimation can be used where only one rebreathing was performed; the line described above is extrapolated to 20 seconds. It should be noted that the PCO_2 is not read at 20 seconds of rebreathing, but a value is calculated by extrapolation (Fig. 6–5).

CALCULATION OF CARDIAC OUTPUT

Because equilibration of CO_2 occurs at a higher PCO_2 in the gas phase than in blood, a correction (the "downstream correction") is applied to the equilibrium (gas phase) PCO_2 to obtain mixed venous blood PCO_2, as discussed previously (p. 60). From the PCO_2 of mixed venous blood and arterial blood the CO_2 content in both sites may be calculated through the appropriate carbon dioxide dissociation curve. Because the rebreathing bag contains about 90 per cent oxygen before the procedure, CO_2 equilibration is with fully oxygenated blood, and the dissociation curve for oxygenated blood is used to estimate venous CO_2 content.

A rapid method for calculating the venoarterial CO_2 content difference was developed by McHardy (1967). His graph (Appendix 2) shows the venoarterial CO_2 content difference for given values of mixed venous PCO_2 and arterial PCO_2 and is constructed for a hemoglobin level of 15 g/100 ml and arterial O_2 saturation of 95 per cent. If these two conditions do not apply, corrections must be made (Appendix 2). This graph also forms one quadrant of a four-quadrant diagram that may be used in the interpretation of results obtained from a Stage 2 test (Chap. 10).

Methods for Blood Sampling

ARTERIAL CATHETER

Although indwelling Riley or Cournand needles can be used for sampling arterial blood during exercise, a small polyethylene or Teflon catheter is better, because it is less likely to cause trauma or become dislodged during arm movements. The brachial or radial artery is used. If the radial artery is chosen, it is wise to precede the catheterization by a simple test to ensure that the ulnar artery is capable of supplying the total blood flow to the hand. This is carried out by compressing both arteries for a short period while the patient exercises his hand, which becomes blanched; the ulnar compression is then released and the skin of the whole hand will flush rapidly if the ulnar collateral supply is adequate.

The catheter can be inserted by the Seldinger technique or with an internal needle. In the Seldinger method (Bernéus et al, 1954), an 18-gauge thin-wall Riley needle is first placed in the artery. Although arterial puncture is a well-established procedure in cardio-respiratory physiology, some details of the technique are worthy of mention. First the artery is precisely located by palpation, and anesthesia of the site is obtained by infiltrating 1 ml of local anesthetic down to the artery. The Riley needle with the obturator half-inserted is then passed through the skin and advanced towards the artery at an angle of about 60° to the surface by a series of small jabbing movements. If the artery is very superficial or mobile it may be stabilized by the index and middle fingers of one hand. On entering the artery, blood will escape around the obturator, which may then be gently pushed home and the needle advanced up the artery for 2 to 3 centimeters; the obturator is removed, and a free flow of blood should be obtained. If blood is not obtained even with the needle tip at sufficient depth, the needle may have passed through both walls of the artery; the obturator is removed and the needle slowly withdrawn until a brisk flow is obtained, when the obturator is replaced. If blood is not obtained on withdrawal, the lateral angle of the needle is changed slightly and then reintroduced. It is important that the needle be well placed in the artery. A flexible nylon or coiled steel guide wire is then introduced through the needle. When the guide wire tip is 15 to 20 centimeters up the artery, the needle is withdrawn over it and replaced by a shaped polyethylene or Teflon catheter attached to a tap; this should pass into the lumen easily, and the guide is then withdrawn. The catheter is filled with heparin-saline and taped to the skin, and the puncture site is covered with gauze and a bandage.

Recently, short Teflon catheters that fit closely over a needle have become available. The needle and catheter are placed in the artery, and when a free flow of blood is obtained, the needle is held and the catheter pushed over it into the artery. The most convenient size is 18 gauge.

The catheters should be filled with a dilute solution of heparin-saline (1000 IU heparin to 500 ml saline) after each sample but may also be continuously flushed with saline under pressure. When the study is complete, the catheter is withdrawn and the artery compressed for at least ten minutes, after which time the compression may be slowly released. The puncture site should be observed for a full minute afterwards to ensure that no leakage is occurring; occasionally compression is required for 20 to 30 minutes. Following compression, it is wise to bandage the site for the rest of the day. If these rules are followed, hematomas will rarely form. However, occasionally a delayed hematoma may appear, leading to extensive skin discoloration 48 to 72 hours after the procedure, but it is usually painless and clears without sequelae. Sometimes arterial puncture is followed by a degree of arterial spasm, identified by diminution in the pulse below the puncture site. However, this is almost invariably relieved within a few minutes by application of heat. Finally, the tips of some fingers may be tender for 1 to 2 days following the procedure; the reason for this is not clear, but it is probably due to platelet emboli.

VENOUS CATHETER

Blood samples for PCO_2, pH, and blood lactate may be obtained from a superficial vein of the warmed hand (Harrison and Galloon, 1965). A catheter similar to those used for arterial sampling is placed in a vein on the back of the hand or just above the wrist. The hand is kept warm throughout the study, using a hair dryer blowing into a plastic chamber which fits over the handlebars of the cycle ergometer, the temperature being kept at about 45° C, or by wrapping an electric heating pad around the hand. The adequacy of arterialization can be checked by measuring the blood PO_2 while the subject is breathing 100 per cent oxygen; if a PO_2 of more than 400 mm Hg is obtained, the blood is adequately arterialized. A PO_2 of more than 80 mm Hg while breathing air may also be taken as evidence of arterialization. This method gives acceptable values for arterial PCO_2 and pH; PO_2 is always underestimated.

CAPILLARY BLOOD SAMPLING

Small samples of arterialized capillary blood may be obtained from the fingertip or ear lobe. Although sampling from either site is not painful, the ear lobe has the advantage of being out of the patient's line of vision. In this technique, a small amount of vasodilating cream such as Trafuril is placed on the ear lobe, and when sufficient vasodilation has been obtained, the lobe is cleaned and swabbed with antiseptic. A small cork is placed behind the ear lobe, and a deep horizontal stab is made with a small pointed scalpel blade in the center of the lobe. During sampling, the site should be kept dry to enhance drop formation and avoid the possibility of contamination by sweat. The best site for fingertip puncture is the side of the middle finger midway in the thickness of the fingertip and just behind the tip, a position close to the digital artery.

Whichever site is used, the capillary blood should be collected into a long capillary tube or into the cup of a heparinized disposable intravenous catheter. If a sample tube of this size (volume of 125 μl or more) is used and flow is brisk enough to fill it within 30 seconds, the measurements of PCO_2, pH, PO_2, and lactate will be close to arterial values (McEvoy and Jones, 1975). However, if flow is not brisk or if manipulation of the ear lobe is required, then the capillary PCO_2 may be a few mm Hg low. It is helpful to have the operator comment on the adequacy of flow and time taken to fill the capillary tubing at the time of sampling.

"FLOAT" CATHETERIZATION OF THE RIGHT HEART

This is a simple procedure, which can be used to obtain pulmonary arterial pressures and blood samples. A nylon catheter (O.D. 0.8 mm) 100 cm long is introduced into the median cubital vein through a wide-bore needle or plastic catheter, or by using the Seldinger technique. A pressure transducer or electrocardiograph electrode is attached to indicate the position of the tip, and the catheter is slowly advanced until it is in the pulmonary artery. The electrocardiograph is monitored continuously. As with classical right heart catheterization, ectopic beats may occur when the tip of the catheter passes into the right ventricle. If ectopic beats occur, the catheter should be withdrawn a few inches and reintroduced. Usually it will float into an adequate position within 10 minutes. Blockage can be prevented by continuous flushing with dilute heparin-saline solution.

Right heart catheterization also may be performed using the balloon catheters of Swan et al (1971), which are, however, of larger external diameter (1.2 mm) and more difficult to introduce percutaneously.

SUBJECTIVE ASSESSMENT OF EXERCISE TOLERANCE

It is helpful to obtain from the patient a description of symptoms during the test. Symptoms may include a normal reaction to heavy work, or an appropriate reaction related to mechanisms disturbed by disease; on the other hand, they may represent an inappropriate reaction to the physiological stress. Frequently a combination of these

TABLE 6–2   RPE SCALE*

6	
7	Very, very light
8	
9	Very light
10	
11	Fairly hard
12	
13	Rather hard
14	
15	Hard
16	
17	Very hard
18	
19	Very, very hard
20	

*From Borg, G.: Perceived exertion as an indicator of somatic stress. Scand. J. Rehabil. Med. 2:92–98, 1970.

factors coexists. Borg (1970) has reviewed these factors and proposed a rating of perceived exertion (RPE) scale, which may be applied in conjunction with exercise testing. The patient is asked to rate the exercise intensity using a symptom score. The numbers chosen for this score (6 to 20) are appropriate for an exercise intensity that in healthy subjects results in a heart rate of 10 times the score. For example, on average the work intensity leading to a heart rate of 170 beats/min is rated "very hard" (Table 6–2). However, the descriptive sentences in the table should be used as a numerical guide rather than a description of perceived exertion: subjects should choose a number on their own scale, where 20 indicates exhaustion.

RECOGNITION AND PREVENTION OF ERRORS

Many tests used in clinical practice are dependent on a single measurement, and quality control is thus relatively simple to maintain. The physiological techniques applied to exercise testing, however, involve many measurements, and accuracy sometimes may be difficult to establish. Furthermore, errors in measurement may compound larger errors in the derived variables. For these reasons, errors should always be looked for, and the techniques should always include routines that will set analytical standards for the test in progress. Although these have appeared already in several chapters, the most important are worth repeating.

Checks Performed at Time of Test

1. The CO_2 analyzer is calibrated at the start and on completion of a test, using at least three gases in the range of 0 to 7 per cent and three in the range of 7 to 15 per cent if rebreathing is to be performed. If more than one sample line is used, calibration should be carried out for each.

2. O_2 analyzers are set up with 100 per cent N_2 as zero and 100 per cent O_2. Air should read 20.93 per cent $\pm$ 0.03 per cent, and it is wise to check the analyzer further by using one of the CO_2 calibrating gases containing about 16 per cent O_2.

3. Analysis of gas with Lloyd-Haldane or Scholander technique. These methods may be used to analyze expired gas collections made in a Tissot spirometer or Douglas bags and are also used to analyze calibrating gas mixtures. Although the "certified" gas mixtures obtained from medical gas manufacturers are usually accurate, they should always be checked.

A surprising degree of error can occur with these techniques. Cotes and Woolmer (1962) circulated a cylinder of gas to several established British laboratories and obtained a variation in O_2 concentration sufficient to cause as much as a 25 per cent error in calculated O_2 uptake. An important check is that air is analyzed accurately ($O_2 - 20.93$ per cent $\pm$ 0.03 per cent; $CO_2 - 0.04$ per cent $\pm$ 0.02 per cent); gas samples are not analyzed until this has been verified. Persistently low (less than 20.90 per cent) O_2 readings indicate that the apparatus or reagents require attention. Repeatability of analysis to within $\pm$ 0.03 per cent is also necessary.

4. Blood gas analysis. Blood gas electrodes are notoriously prone to unsuspected error and are therefore set up using calibrating gases that have partial pressures close to those expected in the samples. Tonometry should be performed regularly, and electrodes should measure the known P_{CO_2} to within $\pm$ 1.5 mm Hg and P_{O_2} to within $\pm$ 2 mm Hg. Wherever possible two blood samples should be taken and analyzed once each; this is preferable to duplicate analysis of one sample.

Periodic Checks

1. Ergometer calibration. Two methods may be used; mechanized and biological. The standard calibration, which should be carried out at least once a year, is obtained by driving the pedals with an electrical or air-driven motor and measuring the torque produced (Cumming and Alexander, 1968). A biological check may be obtained more frequently by measuring O_2 intake at several work rates in one or two members of the laboratory staff. In this method, O_2 uptake should be reproducible to within ±10 per cent at a given power output. If a consistent change is found during such a biological calibration, the ergometer should be recalibrated physically.

2. Dry gas meter. Calibration and linearity should be checked every six months, using a constant volume piston in addition to a check at high flow rates.

3. The respiratory circuit, valves, and taps should be checked for leaks once a week.

Fault Finding

In spite of these checks, errors occasionally occur for several reasons.

1. Gas meter: errors occurring at high flow rates or due to slipping of the potentiometer are easily recognized if ventilation is also measured by a spirometer.

2. Leakage of valves: the most common source is the main two-way valve at the mouth. This may be recognized by a biphasic pattern in the dry gas meter or Tissot spirometer readings and if the tidal gas CO_2 tracing does not fall to zero in inspiration.

3. Incorrect ergometer setting: this is usually recognized by an inappropriate O_2 intake, which may also be an indication that the ergometer needs to be calibrated.

4. Contamination of an expired gas sample with a high O_2 concentration mixture: this is liable to occur following rebreathing and is recognized by high values for the respiratory exchange ratio. It should not occur if criteria for a steady state are observed.

5. Contamination of a blood sample with air: this is likely to occur with capillary blood samples, particularly if flow is poor. It leads to falsely low P_{CO_2} and high P_{O_2} and causes inappropriately low values for the dead space:tidal volume ratio and the alveolar-arterial P_{O_2} difference.

When interpreting results the physiologist should be on his guard against a variety of errors that may result from inaccurate reading of records, faulty calibration of analyzers, and transcription errors. It is wise to recheck any measurement that does not fall within the expected range, by verifying the basic data from the original records. This is particularly important where an abnormal measurement may be of clinical importance. For example, an error in measurement that results in a falsely high mixed venous P_{CO_2} may lead to a calculated cardiac output which is falsely low and on which a clinician may make an important decision regarding the management of the patient.

EXERCISE TESTS FOR SPECIFIC CONDITIONS

Experience has shown that some techniques are of particular value in answering certain clinical problems and should be used in preference to the standardized submaximal tests described above.

Testing for Exercise-Induced Asthma

Exercise-induced bronchoconstriction can be elicited in most asthmatic patients even when they are clinically well. It is also seen in some patients with other types of airway obstruction, such as chronic bronchitis or cystic fibrosis, but in these conditions it is rarely so marked as in asthma.

Exercise testing is valuable in assessing the bronchial lability of patients with asthma and testing the efficacy of various treatments. Running is a more potent stimulus than cycling, and the test is preferably carried out on a treadmill or by "free-range" running on level ground. A work rate sufficient to give a heart rate of about 180/min in children and 150/min in adults should be chosen. A speed of 3 mph (4.8 km/hr) at a gradient of 10 per cent is usually appropriate. If a treadmill is not available, a cycle ergometer Stage 1 test is performed. If bronchoconstriction does not occur it should be tested for following free-range running, in which the patient runs for 6 to 8 minutes in a level, dry, warm corridor at such a speed that he is able to complete the test without stopping. The bronchoconstriction resulting from exercise depends upon the duration of exercise, reaching a maximum after 6 to 8 minutes.

A simple index of airway resistance such as peak expiratory flow rate (PEFR) or one-second forced expired volume (FEV_1) should be measured before the test, and at 1, 5, 10, and 15 minutes after stopping. Usually the fall in these measurements is maximal at approximately 2 to 5 minutes after stopping. There is a slow return to the baseline level during the next 10 to 20 minutes, but a more rapid return can be obtained by an aerosol bronchodilator. Sometimes the bronchoconstriction may begin during exercise, but more commonly its onset is delayed for several minutes after stopping. A nebulized bronchodilator should be available in case of severe reaction. In practice this is rare, but bronchoconstriction remaining 15 to 20 minutes after exercise may be reversed by a nebulized bronchodilator and a further minute of running.

Exercise-induced asthma has been extensively studied by R. S. Jones and his colleagues (1963), who devised a "lability index" calculated on the basis of maximum FEV_1 after a bronchodilator (FEV_{max}), minimum FEV_1 after exercise (FEV_{min}), and predicted FEV_1 (FEV_{pred}):

$$\text{Lability Index} = \frac{FEV_{max} - FEV_{min}}{FEV_{pred}} \times 100$$

Godfrey (1974) has made many contributions in this area, which have helped to define the type of exercise that should be used and the responses in normal and asthmatic children. He suggests that the post-exercise fall in FEV_1 or PEFR expressed as a percentage of the resting value is at least as informative as the lability index. A fall of greater than 10 per cent is considered an abnormal result, obtained in only 5 per cent of nonasthmatic children. A series of studies demonstrated the potency of running compared to other forms of exercise, the relative independence of the percentage fall to the pre-exercise PEFR, and the high (97 per cent) incidence of abnormal responses in asthmatic children and their healthy relatives (32 per cent).

ASSESSMENT OF OXYGEN THERAPY

The issue of portable oxygen therapy frequently arises in patients with severe chronic airways obstruction. Demonstration of improved performance should always precede its regular use. Because such patients usually have extremely limited exercise tolerance, a treadmill is more convenient for testing A speed is chosen which the patient is unable to sustain for longer than three minutes. A study is then performed with the patient breathing from a reservoir of air through a mouthpiece, and the endurance time is measured. The air is replaced with O_2 and the study repeated. Generally a doubling of the endurance time is sufficient evidence that portable O_2 therapy is worthwhile (Cotes, 1963).

Investigation of Ischemic Heart Disease

Although it may seem obvious that an exercise test is of value in the diagnosis of myocardial ischemia, it is in fact difficult to provide documentary evidence of this value, let alone find a generally accepted pattern of investigation and interpretation. Our own experience is not as extensive as that of many other investigators. Although we will attempt to do justice to the vast and recent literature on the subject, this is not the place to attempt a comprehensive review. It does appear that the value of the investigation, in this field as in others, depends on the range and type of experience in the laboratory, and the development of local ground rules governing procedure and investigation. A review of the literature may leave the reader confused. Some studies suggest that an exercise test is almost 100 per cent reliable (McHenry et al, 1972); on the other hand, Redwood and Epstein (1972) believe that there is no evidence to suggest that an exercise test adds any more information than may be obtained from a well-taken history.

Some of the difficulty in interpreting the results of different studies is due to a lack of standardization of procedure and electrocardiographic criteria for a "positive" test. Although procedures vary (e.g., step tests, treadmill, cycle ergometer), it seems unlikely that at a given O_2 intake the choice between these methods leads to appreciable differences in result. Some authorities advise steady-state tests, though again it seems likely that the results are comparable to unsteady tests at a given O_2 intake.

It is generally agreed that several power outputs should be studied, up to a symptom-limited maximum or close to it and that the electrocardiograph should be recorded during, as well as after, exercise. Cahen and co-workers (1973) report a particularly well studied series of 550 patients, in which the exercise protocol was almost identical to the Stage 1 procedure, with the patient exercising to a symptom-limited maximum. Major differences among studies are due in large part to variations in the electrocardiographic criteria used.

ELECTROCARDIOGRAPHIC CRITERIA

There is agreement that the presence of the following criteria is associated with significant narrowing of the coronary arteries, as shown by arteriography, in at least 85 per cent of patients, and that at least 70 per cent of patients with significant arteriographic abnormalities will have abnormalities in the exercise electrocardiograph (Roitman et al, 1970; Cahen et al, 1973; Kattus, 1974).

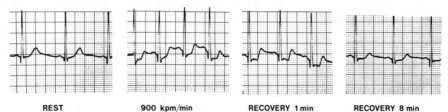

Figure 6–7   Lead V_5 recorded in a patient with ischemic heart disease to show downward-sloping depression of ST segment, beginning at maximal work, becoming more marked early in recovery and resolving rapidly. Note also fusion of T and P waves. Scale: 2 large squares = 1 mv.

1. Horizontal or downward sloping ST segment depressed by at least 0.1 mv for at least 0.08 sec. Some authorities suggest that measurement of the area between the isoelectric line and the ST segment is more objective, in which case the criterion is 0.008 mv sec.

    Lester et al (1967) suggested that measurement of the slope of the ST segment should be related to the extent of its depression, but this method does not appear to be widely used.

2. Inversion of previously upright T wave, when accompanied by ST depression.

3. Increase in T wave amplitude to at least three times the resting value.

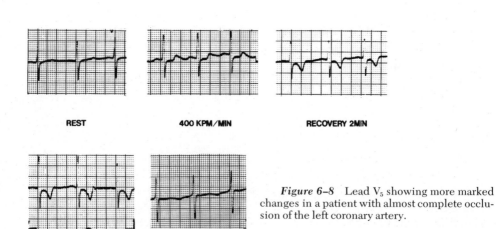

Figure 6–8   Lead V_5 showing more marked changes in a patient with almost complete occlusion of the left coronary artery.

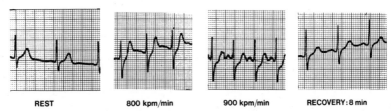

REST   **800 kpm/min**   **900 kpm/min**   **RECOVERY: 8 min**

Figure 6–9   Lead V_4: J point depression developing at 800 kpm/min and becoming associated with ST depression reaching criteria for ischemia and resolving in recovery.

4. ST segment elevation occuring *during* exercise.

A number of related abnormalities are less reliably associated with coronary artery narrowing. ST segment depression to a lesser degree than in Criterion 1 above, upward-sloping depression of the ST segment, and isolated T wave inversion usually are not associated with significant coronary artery disease but should be interpreted with caution. The study may need to be repeated, perhaps with nitroglycerine. If the changes are consistently associated with anginal pain, they are more likely to be significant.

Sometimes these abnormalities evolve into a more characteristic ischemic pattern in the recovery period. Where an ischemic pattern occurs in the recovery period *only,* the earlier it appears and the sooner it resolves, the more likely it is to be associated with significant arterial narrowing. T wave inversion occurring after five minutes of recovery and lasting more than 20 minutes is not associated with significant disease (Cahen et al, 1973). Appearance of negative U wave in exercise in the absence of other signs is an uncommon and inconstant sign of coronary artery narrowing.

Difficulties in Interpretation

In cases where the "isoelectric line" is clearly identified by horizontal isoelectric segments between the P wave and QRS, and between the T or U wave and P wave, there is little difficulty in measuring ST depression and identifying the ischemic pattern.

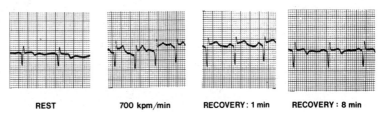

REST   **700 kpm/min**   **RECOVERY: 1 min**   **RECOVERY: 8 min**

Figure 6–10   Lead V_3 recorded in a patient who had suffered a myocardial infarction one year previously: ST segment elevation during exercise.

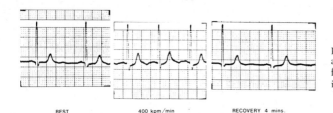

REST   400 kpm/min   RECOVERY 4 mins.

Figure 6–11 Lead V₅ in a patient studied 6 months after acute anterior myocardial infarction; U wave inversion during exercise.

However, during exercise there may be fusion of T, U, and P waves, and the PQ segment may be downward sloping. In addition, during exercise J-point depression with an upward-sloping ST segment is common in normal subjects. These facts often lead to difficulties in ascertaining the presence and the extent of ischemic ST depression (Fig. 6–9).

There are a number of clinical situations which may give rise to misinterpretation.

The "Normal" ST Depression. Depression of the J point with upward-sloping ST segment into an upright T wave is often seen in subjects with healthy coronary arteries and more often in the young than the old. It is not associated with any evolution of pattern and resolves with the heart rate. It does not meet the criterion of 0.1 mv depression for 0.08 sec. Several reports of ST segment depression in normal exercising women that have appeared recently throw further obstacles in the path of the electrocardiograph interpreter (Cumming et al, 1973). The reason for these changes is not clear; in some patients hyperventilation may be the provoking factor. In addition, some healthy subjects show inverted T waves at rest, which become upright during exercise. In cases where this abnormality is found in patients complaining of angina, great care must be taken to obtain a full 12-lead electrocardiograph during exercise, because ST segment changes may be found in other leads (Kattus, 1974).

Vasoregulatory Asthenia. This condition, well described in Scandinavian literature (Levander-Lindgren, 1962), leads to ST segment depression and T wave inversion, which often occurs in

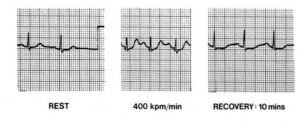

REST   400 kpm/min   RECOVERY: 10 mins

Figure 6–12 Lead V₅ showing fusion of T and P waves and downward sloping P-R segment at 400 kpm/min; delayed depression of ST segment and T wave, not fulfilling ischemic criteria. Recorded in a female patient investigated for effort intolerance, chest pain, and hyperventilation: coronary arteriography normal.

rising from the lying position or during mild exercise but tends to become less with heavier exercise. Furthermore, chest discomfort is not closely related to the appearance of electrocardiographic changes (Friesinger et al, 1972). The cause of the changes is not understood.

Funnel Chest Deformity. Occasionally ischemic ST changes are seen in patients with funnel chest deformity.

Effects of Drugs. ST segment depression during exercise may be seen in patients with patent coronary arteries who are taking digitalis and drugs which lead to hypokalemia.

Most large series (for example that of Cahen et al, 1973) show that an equivocal exercise response will be found in about 5 per cent of patients investigated for angina; in some, the prevention of these changes by pretreatment with nitroglycerine provides supporting evidence of coronary artery disease, particularly if chest pain is improved also.

References

American Heart Association: Exercise testing and training of apparently healthy individuals: a handbook for physicians. New York, American Heart Association, 1972.

Bernéus, B., Carlsten, A., Holmgren, A. and Seldinger, S. I.: Percutaneous catheterization of peripheral arteries as a method for blood sampling. Scand. J. Clin. Lab. Invest. 6:217–221, 1954.

Borg, G.: Perceived exertion as an indicator of somatic stress. Scand. J. Rehabil. Med. 2:92–98, 1970.

Bruce, R. A.: Exercise testing of patients with coronary heart disease. Ann. Clin. Res. 3:323–332, 1971.

Cahen, P., Depouilly, J., Quard, S. and Chazaud, P.: Myocardial ischemia during exercise: electrocardiographic criteria. Data recorded in 553 patients with selective coronarography. Lyon Med. 229:969–980, 1973.

Cotes, J. E.: Continuous versus intermittent administration of oxygen during exercise to patients with chronic lung disease. Lancet 1:1075–1076, 1963.

Cotes, J. E., Davies, C. T. M., Edholm, O. G., Healy, M. J. R. and Tanner, J. M.: Factors relating to the aerobic capacity of 46 healthy British males and females, ages 18 to 28 years. Proc. R. Soc. Lond. [Biol.] 174:91–114, 1969.

Cotes, J. E., and Woolmer, R. F.: A comparison between 27 laboratories of the results of an expired gas sample. J. Physiol. 163:36–37, 1962.

Cumming, G. R., Dufresne, C., Kich, L. and Samm, J.: Exercise electrocardiogram patterns in normal women. Br. Heart J. 35:1055–1061, 1973.

Friesinger, G. C., Biern, R. O., Likar, I. and Mason, R. E.: Exercise electrocardiography and vasoregulatory abnormalities. Am. J. Cardiol. 30:733–740, 1972.

Godfrey, S.: Exercise Testing in Children. Philadelphia and London, W. B. Saunders Co., 1974.

Godfrey, S., Davies, C. T. M., Wozniak, E. and Barnes, C. A.: Cardiorespiratory response to exercise in normal children. Clin. Sci. 40:419–431, 1971.

Harrison, E. M., and Galloon, S.: Venous blood as an alternative to arterial blood for the measurement of carbon dioxide tensions. Br. J. Anaesth. 37:13–18, 1965.

Jones, N. L., Campbell, E. J. M., McHardy, G. J. R., Higgs, B. E. and Clode, M.: The estimation of carbon dioxide pressure of mixed venous blood during exercise. Clin. Sci. 32:311–327, 1967.

Jones, N. L., and Rebuck, A. S.: Rebreathing equilibration of CO_2 during exercise. J. Appl. Physiol. 35:538–541, 1973.

Jones, R. S., Wharton, M. J. and Buston, M. H.: The place of physical exercise and bronchodilator drugs in the assessment of the asthmatic child. Arch. Dis. Child. 38:539–545, 1963.

Kattus, A. A.: Exercise electrocardiography: recognition of the ischemic response, false positive and negative patterns. Am. J. Cardiol. 33:721–731, 1974.

Kelman, G. R., and Nunn, J. F.: Computer Produced Physiological Tables. London, Butterworth and Co., Ltd., 1968.

Lester, F. M., Sheffield, L. T. and Reeves, T. J.: Electrocardiographic changes in clinically normal older men following near maximal and maximal exercise. Circulation 24:5, 1967.

Levander-Lindgren, M.: Studies in neurocirculatory asthenia (Da Costa's syndrome) I, Variations with regard to symptoms and some pathophysiological signs. Acta Med. Scand. 172:665–676, 1962.

McEvoy, J. D. S., and Jones, N. L.: Unpublished observations.

McHardy, G. J. R.: Relationship between the difference in pressure and content of carbon dioxide in arterial and venous blood. Clin. Sci. 32:299–309, 1967.

McHenry, P. L., Phillips, J. F. and Knoebel, S. B.: Correlation of computer-quantitated treadmill exercise electrocardiogram with arteriographic location of coronary artery disease. Am. J. Cardiol. 30:747–752, 1972.

Redwood, D. R., and Epstein, S. E.: Uses and limitations of stress testing in the evaluation of ischemic heart disease. Circulation 46:1115–1131, 1972.

Reindell, H., Konig, K. and Roskamm, H.: Funktiondiagnostik des gesunden und Kranken Herzens. Stuttgart, Georg Thieme Verlag, 1966.

Rochmis, P., and Blackburn, H.: Exercise tests. A survey of procedures, safety and litigation experience in approximately 170,000 tests. J.A.M.A. 17:1061–1066, 1971.

Roitman, D., Jones, W. B. and Sheffield, L. T.: Comparison of submaximal exercise ECG test with coronary cineangiocardiogram. Ann. Intern. Med. 72:641, 1970.

Shephard, R. J.: For exercise testing—a review of procedures available to the clinician. Bull. Physiopathol. Resp. 6:425–474, 1970.

Sjöstrand, T.: A method for the determination of the total hemoglobin content of the body. Acta Physiol. Scand. 16:211, 1948.

Sowton, E., Bloomfield, D., Jones, N. L., Higgs, B. E. and Campbell, E. J. M.: Recirculation time during exercise. Cardiovasc. Res. 4:341–345, 1968.

Swan, H. J. C., Ganz, W., Forrester, J., Marcus, H., Diamond, G. and Chonette, D.: Catheterization of the heart in man with use of a flow-directed balloon-tipped catheter. New Eng. J. Med. 283:447–451, 1970.

Wolmersley, J., Boddy, K., King, P. C. and Durnin, J. V. G. A.: A comparison of the fat-free mass of young adults estimated by anthropometry, body density and total body potassium content. Clin. Sci. 43:469–475, 1972.

Chapter Seven

COMPUTERS IN EXERCISE TESTING

Because of their ability to handle data rapidly, accurately, and on a scale beyond that of other measuring systems, computers are becoming commonplace in respiratory and cardiac laboratories. A computer in an exercise laboratory may be used to calculate and display data, permitting examination and interpretation to take place while the test is in progress. The test procedure may be modified in the light of the results, and the computer may be programed to control some of the testing procedures. These features may be of great value in a busy laboratory, speeding up the processing of results and improving the quality of the tests while at the same time easing the load on the operator. Some of these features will be described briefly.

CALCULATION OF RESULTS

Although a slide rule or calculating machine may be used to calculate results from data obtained in exercise tests, a small digital computer will lead to increased accuracy and speed of calculation, and with some models graphic displays and complex output formats are readily available. The calculations are programed so that only the measurements need be entered, correction factors and constants being automatically applied in the calculations. A program is available which accepts results obtained from a Stage 2 test and displays the limits for arterial PCO_2, cardiac output, and the V_D/V_T ratio, using the logic described in Chapter 3 (Godfrey, 1970).

ON-LINE INFORMATION

Electronic signal conditioning equipment allows the analogue signals obtained from measuring devices such as gas meters and analyzers to be converted into digital form extremely rapidly and accurately. Because the computer can be used to control the measuring processes, the calculation of results is practically instantaneous.

Although the computer need not be located in the laboratory, a terminal in the laboratory is needed to display information and control the selection of computer functions. The results may be presented in alphanumerical form on a printer or oscilloscope, or graphically; information may be stored on a bulk storage device such as magnetic tape, or on a disk unit for later processing. A format suitable for inclusion in hospital charts may be produced, leading to a reduction in secretarial work.

In addition to increasing speed and accuracy of calculations, a computer may be programed to present results in "real time." The results can be examined during the test, so that errors can be detected and decisions made, based on the patient's response. For example, it may become obvious early in a test that the power output is too low to adequately stress the O_2 transport system; the power output may be adjusted according to the heart rate or oxygen intake recorded.

The initial expenditure in terms of time and money has to be considered. Although new technology has significantly reduced the cost of basic computer systems, the associated laboratory equipment, such as gas meters, analyzers, and valves, must be electrically connected to the computer. Development of a program to establish the sequence in which measurements, calculations, and control maneuvers are executed in the test is costly in terms of programing and computer operation. However, several such systems have been developed recently and often it is possible to use the subroutines and programs from these.

At the simplest level, cardiac frequency, ventilation, and breathing frequency are calculated and recorded on line. Addition of automatic expired gas analysis increases the amount of data, and it is at this level that accuracy is improved and time saved. If the expense of a computer is to be justified, the system should be developed to this point at least.

A brief description of the system in use at McMaster University will illustrate the additional equipment required to automate the exercise facility described in Chapter 5 (Fig. 7–1). First, an interface between the input signals and the computer performs analogue-to-digital conversion, signal amplification or attenuation, signal filtering, sensing and recognition of digital inputs, and generation of digital outputs for the control of external devices such as solenoids. Secondly,

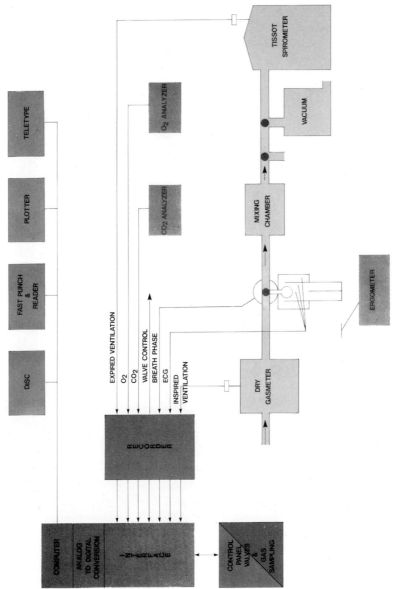

Figure 7-1 Diagram of computer-assisted exercise testing system.

a thermistor at the mouthpiece provides a reference signal to indicate the phase of breathing. Thirdly, a system of sample lines and solenoids sample gas from three sources (the mouthpiece, the rebreathing bag, and the distal end of a mixing chamber or Tissot spirometer). Finally, parallel connection of input signals to both the multichannel paper recorder and the computer allows the use of either or both recording systems. The multichannel recorder system is normally operated in a back-up capacity, when on-line results are obtained on the teleprinter or plotter.

Program development is a major undertaking. Although the work may be reduced by using one of the higher computer languages, this requires a large capital expenditure for peripheral equipment. Assembler or machine language requires only the minimum computer hardware and memory.

The system we have developed is best described by following the procedure used in an exercise test.

1. The operator calls for the exercise program, which is stored in the computer on disk, and the computer first asks for calibrating gas concentrations. The analyzers are calibrated by entering through the teleprinter the composition of two gases of known O_2 and CO_2 concentrations. Each gas is sampled in turn, and the computer uses the results to calculate a calibration factor for each analyzer.

2. Continuing in a question-and-answer mode, the operator inputs the initial work rate and the subsequent increments. In a Stage 1 test, the incremented work level is printed in the data output at one-minute intervals (Fig. 7–2). In a constant power output, Stage 2 or 3 test, the format is altered as the program senses the work rate increment. A zero increment results in a constant work rate test format; any other response results in a progressive Stage 1 test format.

3. The barometric pressure and temperature are entered for use in the gas pressure–volume calculations.

4. A data heading is displayed, and the program enters a pause state. This permits the operator to ensure that the patient is comfortable and that an adequate electrocardiograph tracing is being obtained before the patient begins to exercise. Loadless pedaling is begun.

5. Data acquisition begins, and a time clock starts upon receipt of a simple command on the teleprinter, at the same time that the ergometer load is set.

6. Data are collected and averaged during 20-second periods in the following way. The thermistor at the mouthpiece senses the start of each expiration; the time and initial volume deflection are recorded by the computer for later processing. The CO_2 analyzer

```
INITIAL WORK LOAD   100.,
LOAD  INCREMENTS    100.,
TEMPERATURE 0 C       22.,
BAR. PRESSURE MM. HG.   743.,

INDICATE PLOT OPTION   0.,
```

100 KPM WORK LOAD											
TIME S	HR	VCO2	VE	VT	PETCO2	PECO2	F	VIN	VO2	R	FEO2
.00	1		.00		.0	.0	.0	.0		.00	20.16
.33	77	842	37.60	2422	39.1	20.0	15.5	37.6	898	.93	18.01
.66	74	439	15.08	1208	39.6	26.1	12.4	15.1	524	.83	16.77
200 KPM WORK LOAD											
1.00	75	666	20.28	1402	37.6	29.4	14.4	20.4	760	.87	16.40
1.33	71	602	17.66	1223	38.2	30.5	14.4	17.7	691	.87	16.21
1.66	74		15.31	1540	41.4	.0	9.9	16.2	754	.00	16.12
300 KPM WORK LOAD											
2.00	75	507	14.32	1463	65.2	31.8	9.7	14.4	647	.78	15.58
2.33	72	650	16.30	1836	48.2	35.7	8.8	16.4	784	.82	15.18
2.66	75	593	14.40	1557	43.3	36.9	9.2	14.5	715	.82	15.00
400 KPM WORK LOAD											
3.00	79	675	16.02	1741	44.8	37.8	9.2	16.2	864	.78	14.55
3.33	80	685	16.25	1562	44.5	37.7	10.4	16.5	927	.73	14.24
3.66	83	756	17.27	1556	44.6	39.2	11.1	17.5	990	.76	14.18
500 KPM WORK LOAD											
4.00	82	1034	23.50	1963	45.4	39.4	11.9	XXX	1352	.76	14.15
4.33	84	1144	28.66	2348	41.6	35.7	12.2	28.9	1384	.82	15.16
4.66	85	790	19.09	1830	46.0	37.1	10.4	19.2	949	.83	14.98
600 KPM WORK LOAD											
5.00	88	983	22.60	2057	46.2	39.0	10.9	22.8	1213	.81	14.54
5.33	93	1141	25.65	1915	44.8	39.9	13.3	25.9	1398	.81	14.43
5.66	90	1088	25.08	2441	46.0	38.9	10.2	25.3	1335	.81	14.59
700 KPM WORK LOAD											
6.00	90	1153	25.60	2176	46.1	40.4	11.7	25.8	1383	.83	14.46
6.33	97	1126	24.05	2126	49.9	41.9	11.3	24.3	1365	.82	14.15
6.66	102	1534	34.66	2414	46.7	39.7	14.3	XXX	1858	.82	14.53

Figure 7-2 Segment of computer output obtained in a Stage 1 test.

output is sampled 50 times/sec and the value recorded. At the start of inspiration, the PCO_2 sampled at the mouth falls: this point is recognized by the computer, which stores the highest PCO_2 for the breath being measured ($P_{ET}CO_2$). The 20-second interval is divided into two subintervals to permit measurements of both end-tidal and mixed expired CO_2. End tidal CO_2 is sampled for 15 seconds, and a 5-second interval is allocated for a 2-second measurement of P_ECO_2 and P_EO_2. The electrocardiograph is also sampled 50 times/sec and the R waves recognized and accumulated. At the start of the expiration closest to the end of the 20-second period, time and volume are again recorded, and the breath-by-breath data which have accumulated during the period are averaged.

7. The computer calculates and outputs values of $\dot{V}_I$, f_b, V_T, $P_{ET}CO_2$, P_ECO_2, $\dot{V}O_2$, R, and f_c (Fig. 7–2).

8. The measuring sequence and data averaging continues at 20-second intervals.

9. After $3\frac{1}{2}$ minutes of a constant power output test the computer decides whether criteria for a steady state have been met. Pre-arranged and fixed limits for $\dot{V}CO_2$, $\dot{V}O_2$, $P_{ET}CO_2$, and f_c form the basis for acceptance, and the computer outputs its decision at the end of every 20 seconds. Data are collected for one minute during steady state conditions by an instruction input by the operator (MINC, Fig. 7–3). At this stage the computer uses appropriate data to compute the volume and CO_2 concentration required for the rebreathing gas mixture. The operator applies the information to preparation of the rebreathing bag, using the time-controlled valves described in Chapter 5. The computer is instructed to sample the contents of the rebreathing bag and print the CO_2 concentration as a check.

10. Rebreathing is carried out, and the computer uses the analyzer input to derive mixed venous PCO_2. The operator monitors the

```
.CALL PAGE
.CALL BIN2
INITIAL WORK LOAD    800/.
LOAD INCREMENTS      0.,
TEMPERATURE O C      22.,
BAR. PRESSURE MM. HG.    752.,

INDICATE PLOT OPTION   0.,

800 KPM WORK LOAD
```

TIME S	HR	VCO2	VE	VT	PETCO2	PECO2	F	VIN	VO2	R	FEO2
.00	.00		.00		.0	.0	.0	.0		.00	16.33
.33	117	2359	72.18	3533	42.0	31.9	20.4	72.3	2497	.94	16.36
.66	121	1323	42.32	2057	41.7	30.6	20.5	42.4	1413	.93	16.53
1.00	125	1189	43.89	2061	41.1	26.5	21.2	44.1	1344	.88	16.94
1.33	127	1116	45.58	2066	41.1	23.9	22.0	45.5	1108	1.00	17.68
1.66	129	1711	49.82	2386	41.6	33.6	20.8	49.7	1642	1.04	16.49
2.00	131	1669	47.16	2102	40.9	34.6	22.4	46.9	1493	1.11	16.60
2.33	131	1774	50.14	2208	41.0	34.6	22.7	49.9	1586	1.11	16.60
2.66	135	1966	54.01	2374	40.4	35.6	22.7	53.6	1701	1.15	16.59
3.00	136	1831	51.01	2240	40.0	35.1	22.7	50.7	1591	1.15	16.63
3.33	139	1752	49.50	2081	40.4	34.6	23.7	49.3	1610	1.08	16.50
3.66	140	2031	58.36	2363	39.0	34.0	24.6	58.1	1734	1.10	16.82
4.00	141	1963	59.02	2368	38.3	32.5	24.9	58.6	1678	1.16	17.00
4.33	144	1875	56.38	2238	38.1	32.5	25.1	56.0	1645	1.13	16.92

```
STEADY STATE
BAG DATA: VOL.=3.357   %CO2 = 9.2


EMPTY TISSOT
MINC
```

5.76	147	1893	57.82	2306	37.5	32.0	25.0	57.6	1747	1.08	16.82

Figure 7–3 Computer record obtained during Stage 2 test

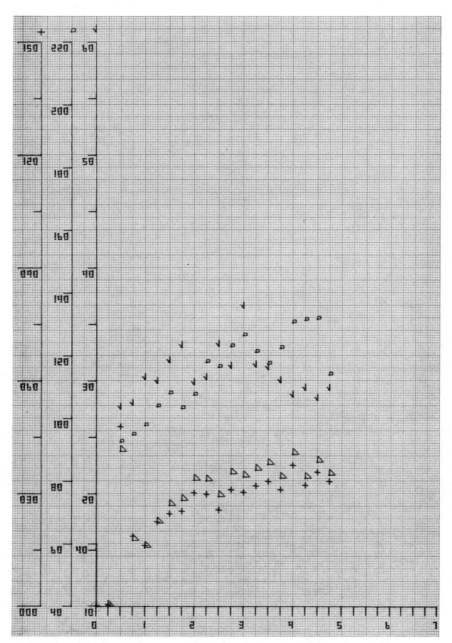

Figure 7-4 Graphical output obtained during a Stage 1 test showing plots of $\dot{V}CO_2$, f_c, $P_{ET}CO_2$, and $\dot{V}_E$ as functions of time.

CO_2 record and decides whether the equilibrium is satisfactory. If the rebreathing equilibrium is accepted by the operator, the computer calculates cardiac output and the V_D/V_T ratio from the measured $\dot{V}CO_2$, P_ECO_2, $P_{\bar{v}}CO_2$, and a value for P_aCO_2 estimated from $P_{ET}CO_2$. If a satisfactory equilibrium was not obtained, the computer uses the collected data to instruct the operator regarding the gas mixture to be used for the subsequent rebreathing.

CONTROL OF THE TEST PROCEDURE

During our development of this system we have learned that there is an optimal balance between automatic control of the procedure by the computer and control by the operator. On the one hand, switching of respiratory circuit and analyzer sampling taps, rapid data collection and processing, calculation of results, and simple decisions regarding the procedure can be made reliably by the computer, freeing the operator to devote more time to the patient. On the other hand, some of the procedural decisions can be made only in the light of the operator's understanding of the patient and his response to the test. The operator must be able to override the computer easily and change the sequence of operations if necessary. Finally, some procedural decisions, such as the quality of the rebreathing equilibrium, are not easy to program and are best left to the operator. In this way the computer can act as a powerful assistant to the operator, allowing him to fully apply his experience in making the test as informative and safe as possible.

A computer can perform several other functions that we have not included in our system but which are well within the capability of a small laboratory computer. It can increase the cycle ergometer load; compare the metabolic response of the patient to that expected for the power output, thus affording a check on the ergometer; automatically mix CO_2 and O_2 for rebreathing; and analyze the ECG wave form to indicate ischemic changes (Rautaharju et al, 1971).

INTERPRETATION OF RESULTS

Because the computer can gather and store data obtained from an exercise test, interpretation of the results would seem a logical extension of its function. Computers are eminently suited to comparing data with established standards and producing a written evaluation or even diagnosis through the use of criteria and limits. In situations where the service load carried by the laboratory is heavy — for example in routine pulmonary function tests (Naimark et al, 1971),

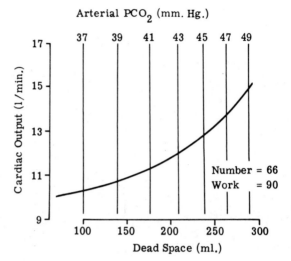

Figure 7-5 Graph constructed by computer to display interrelationships between P_aCO_2, V_D, and $\dot{Q}_t$. (From Godfrey, 1970.)

or for blood gases (Suero, 1970)—the computer can speed the reporting of results without losing any benefit of an expert's opinion. However, exercise laboratories are seldom sufficiently utilized to justify the increased computer storage capacity and additional programing that would be required to handle all the data obtained in an exercise study, and clinical information is always needed for a final interpretation. For these reasons we are currently developing an interpretation program to be applied to data obtained from Stage 1 tests. The more difficult task of interpreting data from Stage 2 and 3 tests will be deferred until experience has been gained with the present system.

In a later chapter we will describe the methods used to establish limits for alveolar ventilation, arterial P_{CO_2}, the V_D/V_T ratio, and the cardiac output, given values of CO_2 output, mixed venous P_{CO_2}, and the mixed expired P_{CO_2} obtained from a Stage 2 test. Godfrey (1970) has detailed a computer program to perform this function and produce a graphical presentation of the relationships (Fig. 7–5). From this graph the limits of these variables are simply defined.

References

Godfrey, S.: Manipulation of the indirect Fick principle by a digital computer program for the calculation of exercise physiology results. Respiration 27:513–532, 1970.

Naimark, A., Cherniack, R. M. and Protti, D.: Comprehensive respiratory information system for clinical investigation of respiratory disease. Am. Rev. Resp. Dis. 103: 229–239, 1971.

Rautaharju, P. M., Friedrich, H. and Wolf, H.: Measurement and interpretation of exercise electrocardiograms. In Shephard, R. J. (ed.): Frontiers of Fitness. Springfield, Ill., Charles C Thomas, 1971, pp. 295–315.

Suero, J. T.: Computer interpretation of acid-base data. Clin. Biochem. 3:151–156, 1970.

Chapter Eight

NORMAL STANDARDS USED IN THE INTERPRETATION OF EXERCISE TEST RESULTS

An exercise test is usually one part of a clinical assessment, the results of which are best interpreted by the clinician himself, or by the clinical physiologist in the light of clinical information. This chapter and those that follow approach interpretation at a series of levels of increasing sophistication, by examining data obtained in patients studied according to the staged procedures described in the preceding chapters. In addition to demonstrating the quality of information obtained from each procedure, the examples will serve to illustrate points made previously regarding the changes in the adaptations to exercise brought about by structural change.

Several problems arise in the interpretation of exercise test results; two will be considered in this chapter. First, there is some variation in measurements made at the same workload, even in the same subject. Secondly, certain factors lead to variation among healthy individuals. Such variation reduces the precision with which the extent of an abnormality may be quantified and may cause difficulty in the recognition of minor abnormalities. Variations due to experimental errors can be kept to a minimum if the test is carefully performed.

123

Errors in the measurement of oxygen uptake and blood gases have been mentioned already.

VARIABILITY IN INDIVIDUAL RESPONSE TO EXERCISE

It may be difficult to know whether the measurements obtained in a test are representative of the patient's usual or his "best" exercise performance. Many factors may influence performance in any one individual, but when formally studied in healthy subjects, the variation in performance has been found to be small. Of course, minor variations in performance by athletes may make the difference between winning and losing a race, but the effect is often trivial when related to performance in submaximal exercise in patients.

Habituation to repeated maximal exercise tests has been found to lead to a reduction in heart rate response (Davies et al, 1970), but the habituation effect is difficult to separate from a training response. Other studies have shown no appreciable effects when exercise tests of the type described in this book were repeated daily in naive subjects (Lane et al, 1974). Anxiety may lead to changes in heart rate and ventilation; these effects may be marked at rest but usually become less during exercise. Shephard (1966) studied the effect of personality in a large group of healthy subjects who exercised on five successive days, and found that anxious subjects were no more variable in their heart rate and ventilatory responses than control subjects. However, hysterical subjects overbreathed in the initial studies, and ventilation became less with repeated testing. Although the majority of healthy subjects who are tested on a cycle ergometer will have comparable results on two successive days, rarely a subject shows an improved performance on the second occasion. Thus it is sometimes necessary to repeat a study on a subject who appears unduly distressed by the test, or who exhibits increased heart rate and ventilation at rest, which remain high throughout the test.

A recent heavy meal influences the metabolic response to exercise and leads to an increase in CO_2 output and ventilation, but again the effect is small (Jones and Haddon, 1973) and easily avoided by performing exercise tests an hour or more after eating.

There is a diurnal variation in the heart rate response to exercise, with lowest levels being found in the early morning (Voigt et al, 1967). Most athletes perform better at this time than later in the day (Conroy and O'Brien, 1973). Although this effect is small, tests should be repeated at the same time of day if changes, either spontaneous or due to treatment, are being studied.

Many drugs are liable to influence heart rate during exercise. Digitalis and propranolol are the most frequently encountered, and results need to be interpreted bearing their effects in mind (Braunwald et al, 1967).

If an attempt is made to avoid these effects, repeated studies at the same power output, carried out on successive days show the following variance in some important variables: oxygen uptake $\pm$ 4 per cent, cardiac frequency $\pm$ 3 per cent, and ventilation $\pm$ 4 per cent (Lane et al, 1974). Such variation should be taken into account in the interpretation of results, and on some occasions a repeat study will be required to identify a minor abnormality.

VARIATION IN PERFORMANCE IN THE HEALTHY POPULATION

It is self-evident that the performance of a small elderly lady cannot be related directly to a standard established in young men attending a college of physical education. Studies in normal subjects have established quantitative effects of various factors, and it is now possible for these to be taken into account in interpreting results, so that a deviation of the observed value from the expected value in the normal population can be quantified more realistically.

Age

The effect of age has been extensively studied. It was shown by Robinson (1938) and later by P.-O. Åstrand (1956) that maximal aerobic power ($\dot{V}O_2$ max) increases during childhood to reach a peak in the late teens, which is maintained until the mid-20s and then gradually declines. The early increase is due to the growth of muscle, heart, and lungs, and the later decline is due in large part to the gradual reduction in maximum cardiac frequency observed with advancing years. Other measurements made at given levels of power output do not appear to be affected by age, if the effects of sex, size, and habitual activity are allowed for.

Sex

Although there are well-marked differences between males and females at comparable ages (Åstrand, I., 1960), these differences largely disappear when other factors such as size (particularly lean body mass) (Cotes et al, 1973), hemoglobin level, and levels of habitual activity are taken into account.

Size

The dimensions of muscles, heart, and lungs influence the response of related mechanisms in exercise, necessitating allowance for the effect of body size. Weight is usually taken into consideration when obtaining the agreed measure of fitness—the maximum oxygen uptake per kilogram of body weight ($\dot{V}O_2$ max/kg). The relevance of this factor to the energy cost of everyday activity is clear (Godin and Shephard, 1973), and it should certainly be considered in relation to the patient's occupation. However, it is not directly related to the performance of O_2 transport mechanisms. A low $\dot{V}O_2$ max/kg in an obese patient may be due to an increase in weight alone and thus may be a misleading value for "the thin man inside, trying to get out," who may have a high degree of cardiorespiratory "fitness." The size of heart, lungs, and skeletal muscle may be poorly related to total body weight, which in this situation is a less reliable predictor of cardiorespiratory performance than lean body mass.

Height is at least as valid an index as weight and in many situations is to be preferred, particularly in children (Gadhoke and Jones, 1969; Godfrey et al, 1971).

Body surface area may appear to be a better index than either height or size, but it suffers from the same disadvantages that apply to weight. Cardiologists usually determine the cardiac index by dividing cardiac output by surface area, and although this may be logical for resting measurements it is of no value for exercise results, where the increase in cardiac output is related to the increase in O_2 intake, body size having little influence (Cotes, 1969).

Fat-free body weight (lean body mass) is reliably obtained from body weight by correcting for body fat, which is estimated from skinfold measurements (Durnin and Rahaman, 1967) or underwater weighing. Measurement of total muscle mass by the radioactive potassium (K40) method is the most reliable index of lean body mass, but it is a time-consuming and expensive procedure. Cotes and his colleagues (1973) have shown that measurement of thigh muscle diameter by radiography is an acceptable alternative. The same group has demonstrated a close relationship between lean body mass and cardiac frequency at oxygen intakes of 1.0 and 1.5 L/min. Thus an index of lean body mass increases accuracy of the cardiac frequency predicted as the normal value at a given power output. This prediction is compared to measurements made in a patient.

Heart Size

Heart size was shown to be related to maximum oxygen uptake by Sjöstrand (1960). The measurement is made relatively simply from antero-posterior and lateral radiographs of the chest and is related to the stroke volume during exercise. It has the added advantage that in patients with heart disease an increase in heart size is accompanied by a reduction in cardiac performance and reduced stroke volume. It seems likely that a measurement of heart volume defines the heart rate response in the normal population, but comparative data with other indices are lacking.

Total Body Hemoglobin

Total body hemoglobin also is related to maximum oxygen intake (Sjöstrand, 1960). In the method which is well established in Scandinavian departments of clinical physiology (Sjöstrand, 1948), a tracer amount of carbon monoxide is rebreathed to obtain equilibration with blood. The same information is obtained from an estimate of lean body mass and the blood hemoglobin level.

Level of Habitual Physical Activity

The level of habitual physical activity influences exercise performance by imposing a degree of "physical fitness." This is an extremely difficult factor to assess, but a measure of the physical activity of patients in their everyday life can be obtained through a simple questionnaire, which allows the observer to categorize patients into four groups: sedentary; sedentary with some daily activity; active, through occupation or recreation activity; and trained athlete.

Race

Race-related differences in exercise performance have been suspected for many years. For example, measurements of $\dot{V}O_2$ max have shown higher values in Scandinavians than in North Americans (Shephard, 1969). Studies carried out recently under the auspices of the International Biological Program have examined performance in different ethnic groups in the Caribbean (Edwards et al, 1972; Miller et al, 1972) and in New Guinea (Cotes et al, 1972). These have shown that there are few race-related differences in exercise performance if allowance is made for variations in size, level of habitual activity, hemoglobin, and altitude of residence.

Measurements of Pulmonary Function

Pulmonary function measurements such as vital capacity, forced expired volume in one second (FEV_1), lung volumes, and carbon monoxide uptake will all show some relationship to exercise performance in the healthy population. However, they are all related to lung size, which is itself related to lean body mass. Although the FEV_1 may be used as a predictor of maximum oxygen intake in health, it is no more precise than other measurements more closely related to lean body mass: this is because ventilation seldom limits exercise in healthy subjects. However, in patients with a ventilatory capacity reduced sufficiently to limit exercise performance, the FEV_1 is a reasonably accurate indicator of maximal ventilation in exercise (Clark et al, 1969).

CONCLUSION

In practice it is simple to obtain measurements of height and weight, and by using three skin-fold thicknesses, lean body mass may also be calculated. In addition, the FEV_1 and VC should be measured. The level of habitual activity can be estimated from data on a simple questionnaire, although a diary card may be required for more precise epidemiological information (Morris, 1973); or the patient may be asked to estimate the greatest daily activity according to Borg's perceived exertion scale (p. 102), which may then be directly related to the assessment made by the patient during the exercise test.

Using the anthropometric data, results obtained in patients may be compared with studies of the healthy population in subjects of the same sex, age, size, and ventilatory capacity, at similar power outputs or at standardized oxygen intakes such as 1.0 or 1.5 L/min. Representative standards are given in Appendix 4.

References

Åstrand, I.: Aerobic work capacity in men and women with special reference to age. Acta Physiol. Scand. Suppl. 169, 1960.

Åstrand, P.-O.: Human physical fitness, with special reference to sex and age. Physiol. Rev. 36:307–335, 1956.

Braunwald, E., Sonnenblick, E. H., Ross, J., Jr., Glick, G. and Epstein, S. E.: An analysis of the cardiac response to exercise. Circ. Res. 20(Suppl. 1):44–58, 1967.

Clark, T. J. H., Freedman, S., Campbell, E. J. M. and Winn, R. R.: The ventilatory capacity of patients with chronic airways obstruction. Clin. Sci. 36:307–316, 1969.

Conroy, R. T. W. L., and O'Brien, M.: Diurnal variation in athletic performance. Proc. Physiol. Soc. September, 1973.

Cotes, J. E., Adam, J. E. R., Anderson, H. R., Kay, V. F., Patrick, J. M. and Saunders, M. J.: Lung function and exercise performance of young adult New Guineans. Human Biology in Oceania 1:316–317, 1972.

Cotes, J. E., Berry, G., Burkinshaw, L., Davies, C. T. M., Hall, A. M., Jones, P. R. M. and Knibbs, A. V.: Cardiac frequency during submaximal exercise in young adults; relation to lean body mass, total body potassium and amount of leg muscle. Quart. J. Exp. Physiol. 58:239–250, 1973.

Cotes, J. E., Davies, C. T. M., Edholm, O. G., Healy, M. J. R. and Tanner, J. M.: Factors relating to the aerobic capacity of 46 healthy British males and females, ages 18 to 28 years. Proc. Roy. Soc. Lond. [Biol.] 174:91–114, 1969.

Davies, C. T. M., Tuxworth, W. and Young, I. M.: Physiological effects of repeated exercise. Clin. Sci. 39:247, 1970.

Durnin, J. V. G. A. and Rahaman, M. M.: The assessment of the amount of fat in the human body from measurements of skinfold thickness. Br. J. Nutr. 21:681–689, 1967.

Edwards, R. H. T., Miller, G. J., Hearn, C. E. D. and Cotes, J. E.: Pulmonary function and exercise responses in relation to body composition and ethnic origin in Trinidadian males. Proc. R. Soc. Lond. [Biol.] 181:407–420, 1972.

Gadhoke, S., and Jones, N. L.: The responses to exercise in boys aged 9–15 years. Clin. Sci. 37:789–801, 1969.

Godfrey, S., Davies, C. T. M., Wozniak, E. and Barnes, C. A.: Ca.diorespiratory response to exercise in normal children. Clin. Sci. 40:419–431, 1971.

Godin, G., and Shephard, R. J.: Body weight and the energy cost of activity. Arch. Environ. Health 27:289–293, 1973.

Jones, N. L., and Haddon, R. W. T.: Effect of a meal on cardiopulmonary and metabolic changes during exercise. Can. J. Physiol. Pharmacol. 51:445–450, 1973.

Lane, R., Jones, N. L. and Kane, J. W.: Habituation to exercise and variation in exercise performance. Unpublished manuscript, 1974.

Miller, G. J., Cotes, J. E., Hall, A. M., Salvosa, C. B. and Ashworth, A.: Lung function and exercise performance of healthy Caribbean men and women of African ethnic origin. Quart. J. Exp. Physiol. 57:325–341, 1972.

Morris, J. N.: Vigorous exercise in leisure time. Lancet 5:333–339, 1973.

Robinson, S.: Experimental studies of physical fitness in relation to age. Arbeitsphysiol. 4:251–323, 1938.

Shephard, R. J.: Initial "fitness" and personality as determinants of the response to a training regime. Ergonomics 9:3–16, 1966.

Shephard, R. J.: Endurance Fitness. Toronto, University of Toronto Press, 1969.

Sjöstrand, T.: A method for the determination of the total hemoglobin content of the body. Acta Physiol. Scand. 16:211, 1948.

Sjöstrand, T.: Functional capacity and exercise tolerance in patients with impaired cardiovascular function. In Gordon, B. L. (ed.): Clinical Cardiopulmonary Physiology. New York, Grune & Stratton, 1960.

Voigt, E. D., Engel, P. and Klein, H.: Daily fluctuations of the performance-pulse index. Ger. Med. Mon. 12:394–395, 1967.

Chapter Nine

INTERPRETATION OF EXERCISE TEST RESULTS

In this and succeeding chapters, we will describe approaches to the interpretation of results. This will be at several levels of sophistication, with the main objective of demonstrating the wealth of information which may be obtained from simple techniques and measurements, using examples extensively. The present chapter deals with the progressive (Stage 1) test; chapters 10 and 11 present an approach to the analysis of results obtained in steady state (Stage 2) tests; chapter 12 uses examples to illustrate the relative values of Stage 1, 2, and 3 tests and to give the reader an opportunity for self-evaluation.

The objective of this chapter is to describe the information available from simple measurements made at many levels of power output up to a maximum level determined by the patient's symptoms or by the criteria established in Chapter 6. The measurements include cardiac frequency, ventilation, and breathing frequency, preferably with O_2 intake and CO_2 output. Properly used, these simple data may allow us to conclude that performance is normal, or, if abnormal, they may provide a quantitative assessment of the factors involved. Identification of the various factors that lead to impaired exercise performance may require further evidence obtained from steady state exercise studies or blood measurements, but even in this situation the information obtained from a Stage 1 test is helpful. The patient is familiarized with the procedure, and the results are used to choose the most appropriate power outputs for study in steady state conditions.

The maximum power output should be examined in relation to sex, age, and size; a convenient way to do this is to convert the power output into an O_2 intake or to use the measured $\dot{V}O_2$ ($\dot{V}O_2$ max). This may be divided by weight to obtain $\dot{V}O_2$ max/kg and compared with established normal values (Appendix 4, p. 201). As indicated in Chapter 8, minor changes cannot be interpreted precisely owing to the many factors which influence $\dot{V}O_2$ max even in healthy subjects.

If results have been obtained at submaximal loads only, the $\dot{V}O_2$ max can be estimated indirectly by extrapolating the relationship between $\dot{V}O_2$ and cardiac frequency (f_c) to a maximal f_c (f_c max) predicted for the patient's age. This practice is hallowed by long usage, and its value in defining $\dot{V}O_2$ max in healthy subjects is well established (Åstrand and Rhyming, 1954; Maritz et al, 1961; Margaria et al, 1965). Using these relationships, $\dot{V}O_2$ max can be predicted to within $\pm$ 12 per cent of the actual value in normal subjects (Davies, 1969). The rather wide variation is due in part to the fact that f_c in some subjects reaches its maximum value asymptotically and also to the variation in maximal heart rates in subjects of the same age.

The "indirect" calculation of $\dot{V}O_2$ max has serious drawbacks when applied to results obtained in patients. Patients with lung disease are often limited by respiratory factors at a $\dot{V}O_2$ well below that estimated from the predicted f_c max. Patients with angina may be limited by pain before f_c has reached a predicted maximum value. Patients with a reduced frequency response due to disease of pacemaker or conducting tissues have an f_c max below that predicted for age. To overcome these difficulties and still obtain a single value that describes the relationship between cardiac frequency and $\dot{V}O_2$, Cotes (1972) has suggested that the relationship be standardized to a $\dot{V}O_2$ of 1.0 or 1.5 L/min. The derived indices, f_c 1.0 or f_c 1.5, were shown by his group (Cotes et al, 1973) to be accurately predicted in a normal population from measurements of lean body mass or thigh muscle circumference. Although such indices are of value in characterizing a group of subjects or patients, in the assessment of the individual patient they are less informative than the complete evolution of the exercise response to power outputs close to maximum.

EXAMPLE 1

We will examine the results obtained in a man of 40 years, weight 85 kg, height 175 cm, Hb 15 g/100 ml, in order to illustrate the factors that should be taken into account in interpreting the results. He achieved a maximum workload of 1400 kpm/min and $\dot{V}O_2$ of 3250 ml/min, 38.2 $\dot{V}O_2$ ml/kg (Fig. 9–1). This is the expected value in an active man (Appendix 4). The heart rate at the maximum load was 190/min; from the relationship of f_c max and age, a value of 210 – (0.65 $\times$ 40), or 184 beats/min, would be predicted. From this we conclude that a maximum heart rate has been achieved and thus may be

EXAMPLE 1   133

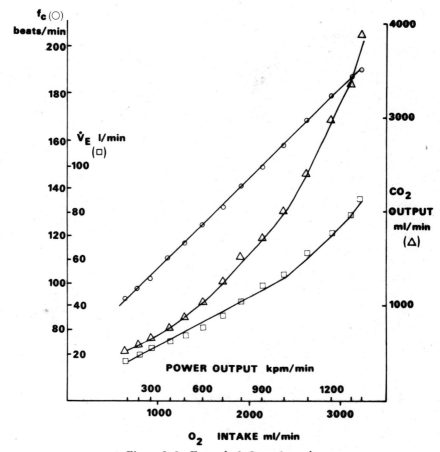

Figure 9–1   Example 1, Stage 1 results.

the limiting factor. Ventilation at the maximum power output was 85 L/min. Sustained ventilatory capacity is calculated from the FEV_1 by multiplying by 35. The FEV_1 was 4.5 liters and thus ventilatory capacity = 157 L/min; we conclude that there is ventilation to spare at the maximum power output and that performance is not limited by his capacity to breathe.

The heart rate response to the multiple power outputs studied is within the normal range for his age. We could leave the interpretation there, but it is more informative to consider the relationship between f_c and $\dot{V}O_2$ using the following logic.

$$\text{Cardiac output} = \frac{O_2 \text{ intake}}{\text{a-v } O_2 \text{ content difference}} \qquad \textbf{Equation 1}$$

$$\dot{Q}_t = \frac{\dot{V}O_2}{C_aO_2 - C_{\bar{v}}O_2}$$

Also

$$\dot{Q}_t = f_c \times V_s \qquad \qquad \textbf{Equation 2}$$

where V_s is stroke volume.
Combining Equations **1** and **2** we obtain

$$\frac{\dot{V}O_2}{f_c} = (C_{\hat{a}}O_2 - C_{\bar{v}}O_2) \, V_S$$

Thus the slope of $\dot{V}O_2/f_c$ depends on the stroke volume, which is relatively constant at levels of $\dot{V}O_2$ above 1 L/min, and the arteriovenous difference. Because there is an effective lower limit to the venous O_2 content, the slope $f_c/\dot{V}O_2$ can give information regarding $V_s \times C_aO_2$. This information becomes more precise if values are obtained at $\dot{V}O_2$ max, when $C_{\bar{v}}O_2$ is at its lowest. Using the lowest value reported in normal subjects and patients (40 ml/L), and assuming an arterial O_2 content of $0.95 \times Hb \times 1.34 \times 10$, we can calculate V_s, the value obtained being the *lowest* value compatible with the results.

Using the example

$$\frac{3250}{184} = V_s \, (190 - 40)$$

$$V_s = 118 \text{ ml}$$

Thus the stroke volume in this subject must be 118 ml or higher.

In studying ventilation we note a linear increase, with $\dot{V}O_2$ up to 2300 ml/min with relative hyperventilation at higher power outputs. This pattern is accounted for partly by an increase in $\dot{V}CO_2$ relative to $\dot{V}O_2$, which is secondary to the production of lactic acid, and partly by alveolar hyperventilation resulting from an associated fall in pH. This pattern of overventilation at high workloads is usually due to anaerobic metabolism as oxygen transport mechanisms reach limiting values and confirms a predominantly cardiovascular limitation.

The normal ventilatory response to exercise up to high levels of O_2 intake suggests normal alveolar ventilation and pulmonary gas exchange. Ventilation also is examined in terms of tidal volume and frequency. The pattern of breathing in this example was normal, with a maximum tidal volume of 3 liters. Thus in this example, a patient referred for assessment one year following myocardial infarction, we may conclude that maximum power output is normal, limited by the cardiovascular system, and associated with normal stroke volume and normal ventilatory response. The electrocardiogram and blood pres-

EXAMPLE 2   135

sure responses to exercise were also normal. From the results we were able to infer normal myocardial function without recourse to complex or invasive procedures, and the overall conclusion is that the response is that of a fit man.

EXAMPLE 2

The results depicted in Figure 9–2 were obtained in a woman 35 years old, height 152 cm, weight 75 kg, Hb 14 g/100 ml. Spirometry showed a VC of 3.50 L and an FEV_1 of 2.40 liters; the FEV_1/VC ratio of 67 per cent indicates minimal airways obstruction.

The maximum power output is well below that in our first example, who was, however, a male patient; in a healthy woman of this age $\dot{V}_{O_2}$ max should be at least 35 ml/kg. It would be unrealistic to multi-

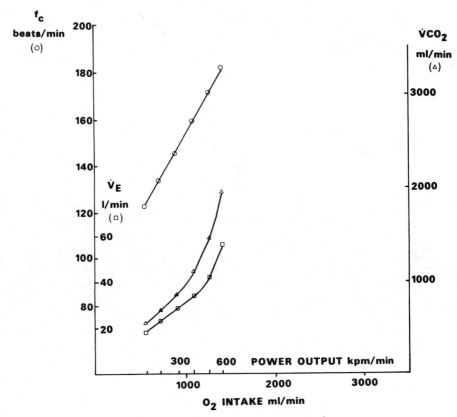

Figure 9–2 Example 2, Stage 1 results.

ply this figure by her body weight, which is well above the ideal weight for her height; skin-fold thickness measurements estimated body fat to be 30 per cent of body weight (i.e., a lean body mass of 52 kg, "ideal" weight 56 kg). Thus her predicted $\dot{V}O_2$ max is 2.0 L/min. Measured $\dot{V}O_2$ at the highest power output (600 kpm/min) was 1.4 L/min. At this power output f_c was 182 beats/min, close to the value predicted for maximal heart rate. Applying the same logic as in the first example, a minimum stroke volume of 51 ml is calculated. This low value is also consistent with the increased slope of $f_c/\dot{V}O_2$; however, it is a *minimum* value—if the a-v O_2 difference is not at a maximum, V_s will be higher.

Ventilation at the maximum power output was 56 L/min. although ventilatory capacity is slightly reduced at 84 L/min (2.40×35), this limiting value was not reached. Ventilation was high throughout the test, with a marked rise at maximum power output; although due in part to a breathing pattern employing high frequency and low tidal volume, a major factor was the increase in CO_2 output. As in the first example this suggests lactic acid production, consistent with a cardiovascular limitation to exercise. This patient was referred for evaluation of breathlessness thought to be due to asthma. The evidence from the Stage 1 procedure, together with an absence of post-exercise bronchoconstriction, suggested that asthma was not the main cause for limited exercise tolerance and that a cardiovascular limitation was predominant. For a fuller evaluation we need information from a Stage 2 procedure (see p. 146).

EXAMPLE 3

The third patient was female, age 31, height 155 cm, weight 51 kg, Hb 14.5 g/100 ml; vital capacity was 3.0 liters, FEV_1 was 1.0 liter; thus the FEV_1/VC ratio is 0.3, indicating moderately severe airway obstruction. Maximum power output was 500 kpm/min, and $\dot{V}O_2$ was 1.25 L/min, well below the predicted $\dot{V}O_2$ max of 1.8 L/min. At this power output f_c was 155 beats/min, below the average maximum value for her age of 190 beats/min. Minimum stroke volume is calculated at 75 ml, and the $f_c/\dot{V}O_2$ relationship is slightly to the left of the average line, suggesting that stroke volume may be somewhat reduced. Ventilation was normal at all power outputs: hyperventilation at high loads was not seen, and at maximum power output, ventilation (34 L/min) was close to the estimated ventilatory capacity of 35 L/min (1.0×35). The pattern of breathing was normal.

The conclusion may be drawn that exercise tolerance is limited

EXAMPLE 3   137

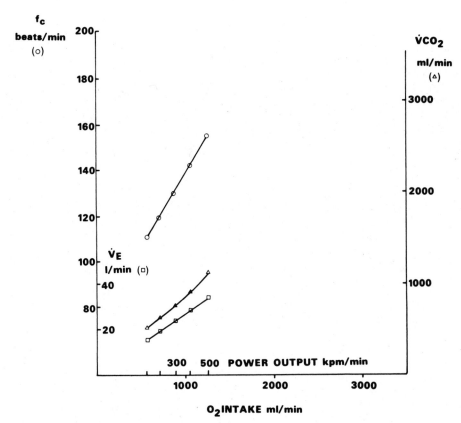

Figure 9–3   Example 3, Stage 1 results.

by ventilatory factors; although a slightly low stroke volume may contribute, cardiovascular factors are not limiting, and anaerobic metabolism is not prominent. The interpretation was helpful in answering the clinical problem "—breathlessness, heart or lungs?" The patient had had a mitral valvotomy many years previously and also had chronic obstructive bronchitis, which was the main cause of her disability.

The Stage 1 test is useful as a screening procedure, providing a simple, rapid, and noninvasive means of establishing whether cardio-pulmonary responses to exercise are normal or not. However, its usefulness is not limited to this purpose alone; quantitative information regarding the severity of cardiac or respiratory malfunction is also obtained, which may contribute to clinical assessment.

References

Åstrand, P.-O., and Rhyming, I.: A nomogram for calculation of aerobic capacity (physical fitness) from pulse rate during submaximal work. J. Appl. Physiol. 2:218–221, 1954.

Cotes, J. E.: Response to progressive exercise: a three-index test. Br. J. Dis. Chest 66: 160–184, 1972.

Cotes, J. E., Berry, G., Burkinshaw, L., Davies, C. T. M., Hall, A. M., Jones, P. R. M. and Knibbs, A. V.: Cardiac frequency during submaximal exercise in young adults; relation to lean body mass, total body potassium and amount of leg muscle, Quart. J. Exp. Physiol. 58:239–250, 1973.

Davies, C. T. M.: Measuring the fitness of a population. Proc. R. Soc. Med. 62:1171–1174, 1969.

Margaria, R., Aghemo, P. and Rovelli, E.: Indirect determination of maximal O_2 consumption in man. J. Appl. Physiol. 20:1070–1073, 1965.

Maritz, J. S., Morrison, J. F., Peter, J., Strydom N. B. and Wyndham, C. H.: A practical method of estimating an individual's maximum oxygen intake. Ergonomics 4: 97–122, 1961.

Chapter Ten

INTERPRETATION

A FOUR-QUADRANT DIAGRAM FOR USE IN THE INTERPRETATION OF TESTS

> Let me commence by drawing your attention to four sets of measurements which will be considered at first quite separately, but which later will prove not to be so unconnected as might appear at first sight.

With these words Sir Joseph Barcroft (1934) introduced the reader of *Features in the Architecture of Physiological Function* to the adaptation to exercise, considered as a series of four equations describing oxygen transport. As was first shown by Murray and Morgan (1925), the graphical display of these equations may be combined in a diagram having four quadrants. The resulting chart was used by Barcroft to explore the interrelationships between mechanisms in order to define their limits and the extent of their capacity to adapt to an increase in metabolism.

We will perform a similar task related to the transport of CO_2 from tissues to expired gas. In addition to describing graphically the mechanisms and their interrelationship, the diagram lends itself to use as a teaching tool by giving insight into the mechanisms involved. It may also be used in the calculation and interpretation of exercise tests.

The four equations used have been noted previously and are repeated here in order to describe the construction of the diagram.

Mixed expired P_{CO_2} expresses the ventilatory response to an increase in CO_2 output.

$$P_E CO_2 = \frac{\dot{V}_{CO_2} \times 0.863}{\dot{V}_E}$$

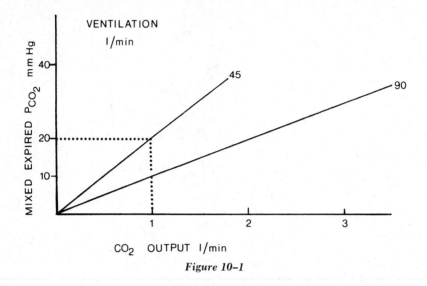

Figure 10–1

This relationship is described by a graph having CO_2 output as the abscissa and P_ECO_2 as the ordinate, and in which a family of isopleths for ventilation is drawn.

Notice that for a given $\dot{V}CO_2$ (1 L/min in the example shown in Fig. 10–1), doubling ventilation (from 45 to 90 L/min) leads to a halving of P_ECO_2 (from 20 to 10 mm Hg).

Total expired ventilation ($\dot{V}_E$) has two components—alveolar ventilation ($\dot{V}_A$), and dead space ventilation ($\dot{V}_D$). The mixed expired PCO_2 at any given CO_2 output is related to $\dot{V}_A$ and the V_D/V_T ratio through the following series of equations:

$$\dot{V}_A = \frac{\dot{V}CO_2 \times 0.863}{P_aCO_2}$$

and

$$V_D/V_T = \frac{P_aCO_2 - P_ECO_2}{P_aCO_2} \qquad \textbf{(Bohr's equation)}$$

Thus at a given $\dot{V}CO_2$, $\dot{V}_A$ influences both P_aCO_2 and the absolute difference between P_aCO_2 and P_ECO_2. Therefore a low P_ECO_2 may be due to an increase in $\dot{V}_A$ or V_D/V_T, or both.

From Bohr's equation

$$P_ECO_2 = P_aCO_2 (1 - V_D/V_T)$$

or

$$P_E CO_2 = \frac{\dot{V}CO_2 \times 0.863}{\dot{V}_A} (1 - V_D/V_T)$$

We may construct a graph having $P_E CO_2$ as the ordinate and $P_a CO_2$ as the abscissa, and in which isopleths of V_D/V_T ratio are drawn.

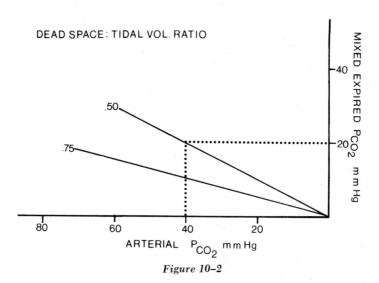

Figure 10-2

In Figure 10–2, $P_E CO_2$ is 20 mm Hg, $P_a CO_2$ is 40 mm Hg, and V_D/V_T is 0.5. Notice that the higher the value for V_D/V_T, the greater the difference between $P_a CO_2$ and $P_E CO_2$, but also that for a given V_D/V_T ratio this difference becomes smaller if $P_a CO_2$ falls, that is, if alveolar ventilation increases.

The process of CO_2 carriage by blood is described by the dissociation curve relating CO_2 content to CO_2 pressure. Because we are concerned with both venous and arterial blood there are logical and mathematical arguments for expressing this process as the relationship between the venoarterial pressure *difference* and the venoarterial content *difference:*

$$(C_{\bar{v}} CO_2 - C_a CO_2) = f (P_{\bar{v}} CO_2 - P_a CO_2)$$

where f is a function of the CO_2 dissociation curve. The advantage of this approach, introduced by McHardy (1967), is that absolute CO_2

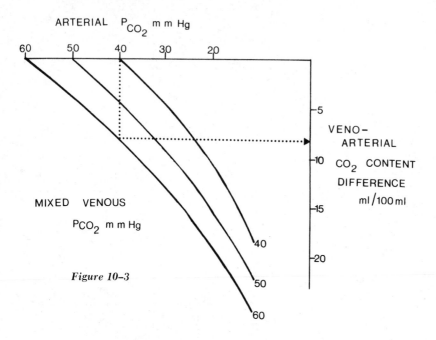

ARTERIAL P_{CO_2} m m Hg

VENO–
ARTERIAL
CO_2 CONTENT
DIFFERENCE
ml / 100 ml

MIXED   VENOUS
P_{CO_2} m m Hg

Figure 10–3

content need not be derived from the separate values of $P_{\bar{v}}CO_2$ and P_aCO_2, which simplifies graphical plotting of data.

This relationship may be plotted with P_aCO_2 as the abscissa and the venoarterial CO_2 content difference as the ordinate. The CO_2 dissociation curve may then be used to construct a series of curved lines, which are isopleths of $P_{\bar{v}}CO_2$. The lines are constructed for an arterial O_2 saturation of 95 per cent and mixed venous O_2 saturation of 100 per cent, so that the curves, which have been derived for blood of hemoglobin content 15 g/100 ml, may be used for oxygenated $P_{\bar{v}}CO_2$ measured by rebreathing. Deviations from this arterial O_2 saturation or hemoglobin content influence the relationships, and corrections are made to the CO_2 content difference to allow for them.

The example shows that for P_aCO_2 of 40 mm Hg and $P_{\bar{v}}CO_2$ of 60 mm Hg, the CO_2 content difference is 8.4 ml/100 ml.

At any CO_2 output, the venoarterial content difference is governed by the cardiac output. This is expressed mathematically using the Fick principle.

$$\dot{Q}_t = \frac{\dot{V}CO_2}{C_{\bar{v}}CO_2 - C_aCO_2}$$

This is expressed conveniently by a graph having $\dot{V}CO_2$ as the abscissa and $(C_{\bar{v}}CO_2 - C_aCO_2)$ as the ordinate, with isopleths of $\dot{Q}_t$ radiating from their intersection.

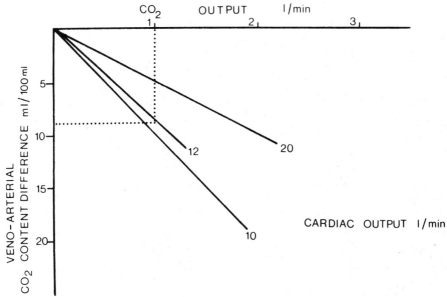

Figure 10–4   At a CO_2 output of 1 L/min, a v̄-a difference of 8.4 ml indicates cardiac output is 12 L/min.

Each of these relationships describes a portion of the CO_2 transport system. We may now combine the four graphs to obtain a single figure that allows us to solve the equations, given data obtained in an exercise test (Fig. 10–5) (McHardy et al, 1967).

In the example used above to illustrate the construction of the diagram, all the values necessary to calculate V_D/V_T, $\dot{V}_A$, and $\dot{Q}_t$ were given; that is, $\dot{V}CO_2$, P_ECO_2, P_aCO_2, and $P_{\bar{v}}CO_2$. The main function of the diagram is to explore the limits of these interrelated variables where P_aCO_2 is not measured. Therefore, in the examples which follow, the data will be analyzed initially without benefit of the blood data. This will allow the reader to judge the value of the data collected in Stage 2 and Stage 3 procedures. Although data are usually recorded at more than one power output, the analysis will be limited to one for the sake of brevity. The first example will use data obtained from the first patient in the previous chapter.

Example 1

Male, age 40 (Example 1, Chapter 9)

Power Output kpm/min	w	f_c beats/min	f_b breaths/min	$\dot{V}CO_2$ ml/min	P_ECO_2 mm Hg	$P_{\bar{v}}CO_2$ mm Hg
800	133	145	20	2000	36	70

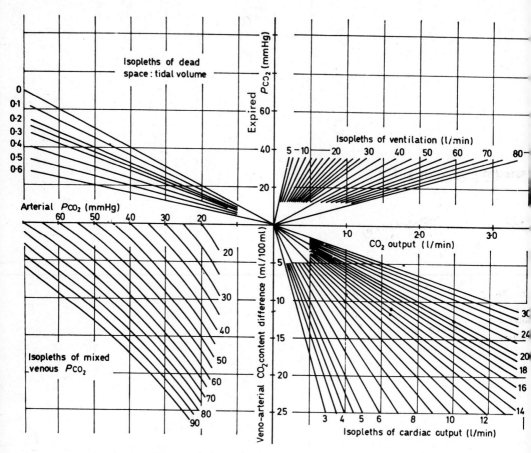

Figure 10–5   McHardy's four-quadrant diagram.

Starting in the upper right hand quadrant, P_ECO_2, which lies on the ventilation isopleth of 48 L/min, is plotted. A horizontal line is drawn into the upper left quadrant until the isopleth representing the lowest limit of V_D/V_T is met. The lowest value is chosen from the normal values for adults, given in Chapter 2; for children a value may be predicted from the patient's height, using the nomogram of Radford (1954).

In the example, the tidal volume is 2400 ml, and the lowest value for the dead space volume, including an instrumental dead space of 60 ml, is 240 ml, giving a V_D/V_T ratio of 0.10 (Jones et al, 1966) (Point 1 in Fig. 10–6). Dropping a vertical line from the intersection P_ECO_2 36, V_D/V_T 0.10 meets the P_aCO_2 abscissa at 40 mm Hg (Point 2). The vertical line is continued down to the $P_{\bar{v}}CO_2$ isopleth, and a horizontal line from this intersection meets the venoarterial CO_2 content

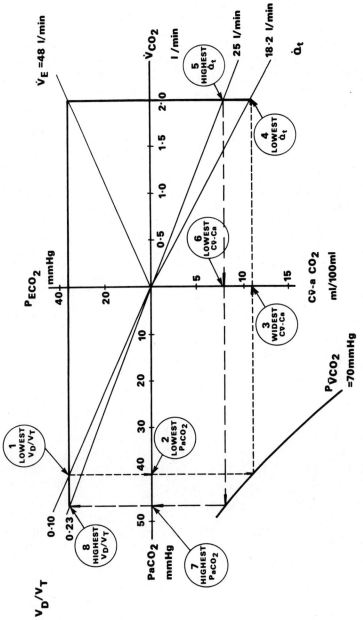

Figure 10-6   Example 1: analysis of Stage 2 results.

difference ordinate at 11.0 ml/100 ml (Point 3). Corrections would need to be applied for hemoglobin values above or below 15 g/100 ml and for arterial O_2 desaturation. Continuing the line into the fourth quadrant to intersect a line dropped from the $\dot{V}CO_2$ yields a cardiac output of 18.2 L/min (Point 4). Note that by choosing the *lowest* value for V_D/V_T we obtained the *lowest* value for P_aCO_2, *highest* value for $C_{\bar{v}\text{-}a}CO_2$, and *lowest* value for $\dot{Q}_t$. We may conclude that the lowest stroke volume is 125 ml (18,200 ÷ 145).

By going round the diagram in an opposite direction we can test the data further to obtain highest values for P_aCO_2 and V_D/V_T. The starting point is defined by choosing the highest likely value for V_s. Using an estimate of 175 ml, the appropriate cardiac output is 25 L/min (175 × 145) (Point 5). Moving horizontally to the left from the intersection of the $\dot{Q}_t$ isopleth and the vertical line dropped from $\dot{V}CO_2$, a value for $C_{\bar{v}\text{-}a}CO_2$ of 8.0 ml/100 ml is obtained (Point 6): the line is extended to the $P_{\bar{v}}CO_2$ isopleth and extended vertically to obtain a PCO_2 of 47 mm Hg (Point 7) and V_D/V_T of 0.23 (Point 8). This is the highest value compatible with the data, but is still within normal limits.

Without blood values we may conclude that P_aCO_2 is 40 to 47 mm Hg, V_D/V_T is 0.10 to 0.23, and $\dot{Q}_t$ equals 18 to 25 L/min. Thus although P_aCO_2 was measured in this study at 43.0 mm Hg, it was not required to establish that the responses to exercise were normal.

Example 2

Female, age 35 (Example 2, Chapter 9)

Power Output kpm/min	w	f_c beats/min	f_b breaths/min	$\dot{V}CO_2$ ml/min		P_ECO_2 mm Hg	$P_{\bar{v}}CO_2$ mm Hg
400	67	168	30	1340	1120	22.3	65

Analyzing the data in the same manner as for Example 1 we obtain the following solutions:

Lowest V_D/V_T	P_aCO_2	$C_{\bar{v}\text{-}a}CO_2$	Lowest $\dot{Q}_t$
0.15	26	17.0	7.8

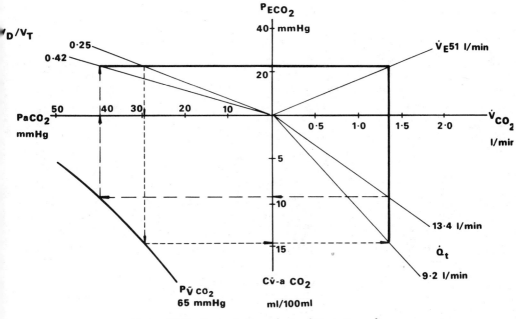

Figure 10-7   Example 2: analysis of Stage 2 results.

Highest V_s	Highest $\dot{Q}_t$	$C_{\bar{v}\text{-}a}CO_2$	P_aCO_2	Highest $\dot{V}_D/V_T$
125	21.0	6.4	48	0.53

The limits defined are wider than in the first example, and it is not possible to conclude that the values *must* lie within normal limits.

Another set of solutions may be chosen as follows to determine whether the results *could* be within normal limits (Fig. 10-7).

Highest V_D/V_T	P_aCO_2	$C_{\bar{v}\text{-}a}CO_2$	Is $\dot{Q}_t$ normal?
0.25	30	14.5	9.2

Lowest V_s	$\dot{Q}_t$	$C_{\bar{v}\text{-}a}CO_2$	P_aCO_2	Is V_D/V_T normal?
80	13.4	10	39	0.42

The four-quadrant diagram allows this solution to be tested rapidly, and it is apparent that the values cannot be fitted to any normal solution. The highest value for $\dot{Q}_t$ compatible with normal V_D/V_T is 9.2 L/min, which is below the normal range. This implies a V_S of only 54 ml. A normal value for V_S, however, implies a high V_D/V_T. The unique solution, given by a measurement of P_aCO_2, can be approached by estimating P_aCO_2 from $P_{ET}CO_2$. $P_{ET}CO_2$ was 33 mm Hg, and estimated P_aCO_2 was 32 mm Hg, suggesting both a low cardiac output and increased V_D/V_T.

In many situations this information will be sufficient to answer the clinical question; however, if blood gas measurements are available, the uncertainty may be eliminated. P_{CO_2} measured in capillary blood was 34 mm Hg, the derived values being $V_D/V_T = 0.34$ and $\dot{Q}_t = 10.7$ L/min. Stroke volume was 63 ml, a reduced value, and physiological dead space 450 ml, which is increased. The data obtained in this procedure confirm the conclusion drawn from the Stage 1 test (Example 2 in the previous chapter) — that the cardiac response to exercise was abnormal — but also give more quantitative information regarding the disturbance, and permit detailed analysis of the ventilatory response. The combination of reduced stroke volume, alveolar hyperventilation, and increased V_D/V_T ratio is compatible with pulmonary vascular obstructive disease, a diagnosis confirmed later by cardiac catheterization.

Example 3

Female, age 31 (Example 3, Chapter 9)

Power Output kpm/min w	f_c beats/min	f_b breaths/min	$\dot{V}CO_2$ ml/min	$\dot{V}O_2$ ml/min	P_ECO_2 mm Hg	$P_{\bar{v}}CO_2$ mm Hg
300 50	136	25	1060	940	32	83

As in Example 2, starting with the lowest possible V_D/V_T and highest possible $\dot{Q}_t$ does not yield solutions in which all variables *must* be normal. Again, we test the data to see if normal values *can* be obtained.

Highest V_D	V_D/V_T	P_aCO_2	$C_{\bar{v}-a}CO_2$	$\dot{Q}_t$
200 ml (+60 ml)	0.23	41.5	14.5	7.3

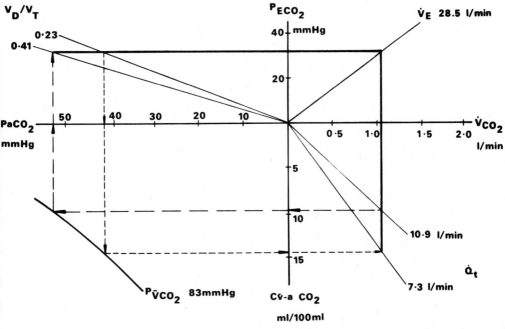

Figure 10–8   Example 3: analysis of Stage 2 results.

Lowest $\dot{Q}_t$	$C_{\bar{v}\text{-}a}CO_2$	P_aCO_2	V_D/V_T	V_D
10.9	9.7	53.5	0.41	400

Neither alternative leads to a normal solution, and again we need P_aCO_2 to obtain unique values. End tidal PCO_2 was 51 mm Hg, suggesting that the second is closer to the true values than the first. The interpretation is that ventilatory impairment is the major abnormality, leading to increased V_D/V_T ratio and alveolar underventilation; note, however, that $\dot{V}_E$ was normal at 28.5 L/min. Cardiac output is probably normal also. P_aCO_2 cannot be estimated accurately from end tidal PCO_2 if severe airway obstruction is present, but an approximation may be obtained. Arterial PCO_2 in this patient was 52 mm Hg, confirming the diagnosis of alveolar underventilation, increased V_D/V_T ratio (0.33), and normal cardiac output (10.3 L/min) with slightly low stroke volume (76 ml).

OTHER USES OF THE DIAGRAM

In this chapter we have described the use of the four-quadrant diagram in interpreting data obtained from a bloodless exercise procedure, the Stage 2 test. Although the diagram was both a product of and a stimulus to the development of this approach to exercise testing, we would not wish to leave the impression that it is merely an analogue computer for the calculation of results. Since its design nearly a decade ago its main role has gradually changed.

Of course, its function as a computer is easily replaced by a digital computer programed to derive results more rapidly and more accurately. At the next level— and this is where its value was greatest in the developmental phase—the diagram is used to set limits to possible combinations of alveolar ventilation, V_D/V_T ratio, and cardiac output, given measurements of CO_2 output, $P_{\bar{v}}CO_2$, and P_ECO_2 obtained in a Stage 2 procedure. This feature, described in the present chapter, may also be performed by a computer (Godfrey, 1970).

There is a third level at which we think the diagram is still unique. This is in its use as a teaching device to gain physiological insight into the quantitative interaction of variables adapting to the demands of exercise. It provides a grasp of the physiological architecture that supports the transport of O_2 and CO_2, in a similar manner to a diagram used by Barcroft (1934) to depict O_2 transport. Barcroft credits Murray and Morgan (1925) with the first demonstration of the importance of such a diagram, which emphasized the value of assessing cardiorespiratory function through the stress of an increased oxygen load, in the same way that our diagram uses CO_2. By making use of the interdependence between physiological mechanisms, the diagram also illuminates the often paradoxical situation in which analytical accuracy may have little physiological significance and vice-versa.

To emphasize these points we will consider examples taken from each of the four quadrants.

Quadrant 1 — The Ventilation Quadrant

Physiologically, contrast the difference in ventilation required to lower expired P_{CO_2} from 30 to 20 mm Hg, at CO_2 outputs of 0.5 L/min and 2 L/min. At 0.5 L/min $\dot{V}_{CO_2}$ the difference in ventilation is only 6 L/min; at 2 L/min $\dot{V}_{CO_2}$ it is 30 L/min. In a patient with limited ventilatory reserve a change in ventilation of this order may have a striking effect on respiratory work, a quadratic function of ventilation, leading to an increase in the total oxygen demand.

Analytically, note the unimportance of accuracy in measurement of $\dot{V}_{CO_2}$ at levels around 0.5 L/min and the accuracy required at 2.0

L/min: if $\dot{V}_E$ is assumed to be accurate, ± 5 mm Hg variation in the measurement of P_ECO_2 leads to ± 46 ml in $\dot{V}CO_2$ at a $\dot{V}CO_2$ of 0.5 L/min, but to ± 320 ml in $\dot{V}CO_2$ at a $\dot{V}CO_2$ of 2.0 L/min.

Quadrant 2 – The Dead Space Quadrant

Physiologically, contrast the difference in arterial P_{CO_2} caused by an increase in the V_D/V_T ratio from 0.1 to 0.2 (4 mm Hg) to that caused by an increase from 0.5 to 0.6 (10 mm Hg), at values of P_aCO_2 around 40 mm Hg. Also contrast the effect on P_aCO_2 of an increase in V_D/V_T from 0.1 to 0.2 at a P_ECO_2 of 20 mm Hg (+ 2 mm Hg) to that at a P_ECO_2 of 40 mm Hg (+6 mm Hg).

Analytically, note the unimportance of accuracy in P_aCO_2 when the V_D/V_T ratio is high compared to the accuracy required at normal V_D/V_T. At a P_ECO_2 of 20 mm Hg, a 2 mm Hg error in P_aCO_2 leads to a doubling of V_D/V_T from a true value of 0.1 to 0.2: the same error results in an increase in V_D/V_T of only 0.02 when the true value is 0.5.

Quadrant 3 – The CO_2 Dissociation Curve

Physiologically, contrast the pressure difference required to transport 10 ml CO_2/100 ml when P_aCO_2 is 35 mm Hg to that when P_aCO_2 is 50 mm Hg, 20 mm Hg in the first instance compared to 30 mm Hg in the second.

Analytically, contrast the relative importance of an error in the $P_{\bar{v}}CO_2$-P_aCO_2 difference at low P_{CO_2} compared with the effect at high P_{CO_2}. An overestimate of 2 mm Hg in a 30 mm Hg pressure difference will increase figures for venoarterial content by 1.6 ml/100 ml when $P_{\bar{v}}CO_2$ is 50 mm Hg and by 0.8 ml/100 ml when $P_{\bar{v}}CO_2$ is 80 mm Hg.

Quadrant 4 – The Fick Cardiac Output Quadrant

Physiologically, note that if $\dot{Q}_t$ is unable to increase to more than 10 L/min, a $\dot{V}CO_2$ level of 1 L/min may easily be achieved at a venoarterial difference of 10 ml/100 ml. However, a CO_2 of 2 liters cannot be sustained, because an a-v difference of 20 ml/100 ml would be required.

Analytically, contrast the error in the estimate of cardiac output produced by miscalculation of 1 ml/100 ml in the venoarterial CO_2 content difference at a $\dot{V}CO_2$ of 0.5 L/min (difference in $\dot{Q}_t$ of 0.5 L/min) and at 2 L/min (a difference of 2 L/min).

THE FOUR QUADRANTS COMBINED

Finally, all four quadrants may be put to use. *Physiologically,* note the relative stress on the CO_2 transport mechanisms in maintaining a CO_2 output of 1.5 L/min in a patient with chronic airway obstruction and severe gas exchange disturbance, which leads to a V_D/V_T ratio of 0.5. If alveolar ventilation is maintained and P_aCO_2 kept at 40 mm Hg, mixed venous PCO_2 will be 70, expired PCO_2 will be 20, and thus a ventilation of 65 L/min is required. If alveolar underventilation is "accepted" by the system, with an arterial PCO_2 of 60 mm Hg, mixed venous PCO_2 is then 95 mm Hg, mixed expired PCO_2 is 30 mm Hg, and ventilation is 42 L/min. When the difference in ventilation is considered in relation to reduced ventilatory capacity and increased respiratory work, the effect is magnified. Finally, consider the effect of a limited cardiac reserve in such a patient: if maximum cardiac output is 10 L/min, a CO_2 output of 1.5 L/min may be maintained only if alveolar ventilation is capable of maintaining P_aCO_2 at 45 mm Hg or less, without the mixed venous PCO_2 rising to above 90 mm Hg. A rise in PCO_2 of this degree will be paralleled by a rise in tissue PCO_2 and thus of hydrogen ion concentration. In this way the diagram can illustrate the extent to which the internal environment is affected by changes in the capacities of the CO_2 and O_2 transport mechanisms as they adapt to the demands imposed by the increased metabolism of exercise.

Analytically, consider the effect of a 2 mm Hg error in the measurement of arterial PCO_2 on the calculated cardiac output at a $\dot{V}CO_2$ of 1.5 L/min if true P_aCO_2 is 25 mm Hg (error in $\dot{Q}_t$ is 1.9 L/min), 40 mm Hg (error is 1.5 L/min), or 55 mm Hg (error is 0.9 L/min).

References

Barcroft, J.: Features in the Architecture of Physiological Function. Cambridge University Press. Reprinted by Hafner Publishing Co., New York, 1972.

Godfrey, S.: Manipulation of the indirect Fick principle by a digital computer program for the calculation of exercise physiology results. Respiration 27:513–532, 1970.

Jones, N. L., McHardy, G. J. R., Naimark, A. and Campbell, E. J. M.: Physiological dead space and alveolar-arterial differences during exercise. Clin. Sci. *31*:19–29, 1966.

McHardy, G. J. R.: Relationship between the difference in pressure and content of carbon dioxide in arterial and venous blood. Clin. Sci. *32*:299–309, 1967.

McHardy, G. J. R., Jones, N. L. and Campbell, E. J. M.: Graphical analysis of CO_2 transport. Clin. Sci. *32*:289–298, 1967.

Murray, C. E., and Morgan, J.: Oxygen exchange, blood, and the circulation. A coordinated treatment of the factors involved in oxygen supply on the basis of the diffusion theory. J. Biol. Chem. *65*:419–444, 1925.

Radford, E. P.: Ventilation standards for use in artificial respiration. J. Appl. Physiol. *7*:450–451, 1954–55.

Chapter Eleven

INDIRECT ESTIMATION OF LACTIC ACID PRODUCTION IN BLOODLESS EXERCISE TESTS

Production of lactic acid by muscle is an indication that anaerobic metabolic pathways are being used in muscle and thus that oxygen supply is not keeping pace with demand. Lactic acid reacts with bicarbonate in tissue fluids and induces the formation of carbonic acid, increasing the production of CO_2 in the body. Most of this CO_2 will be excreted with CO_2 from aerobic metabolism, leading to an increased CO_2 output in the lungs and to a high value for the respiratory exchange ratio (R). Various approaches have been used to estimate lactic acid accumulation from measurements of R (Issekutz et al, 1962; Naimark et al, 1964). However, during exercise, a variable amount of CO_2 is accumulated in body stores and is not excreted into expired gas. Thus more accurate estimates of lactic acid production are obtained from measurements of expired CO_2 and mixed venous P_{CO_2} by constructing a CO_2 balance equation having four components.

$$\text{Total } CO_2 \text{ output} = CO_2 \text{ produced by aerobic metabolism}$$
$$\pm\ CO_2 \text{ moving into or out of stores}$$
$$+\ CO_2 \text{ resulting from lactic acid production}$$

$$\text{Total } \dot{V}_{CO_2} = \text{aerobic } \dot{V}_{CO_2} \pm \text{ stored } CO_2 + CO_2 \text{ (lactic acid)}$$
$$\quad 1 \qquad\qquad 2 \qquad\qquad 3 \qquad\qquad 4$$

1 is measured.

2 is calculated from $\dot{V}O_2$ by assuming a value for the R.Q. in muscle.

3 is calculated from changes in $P_{\bar{v}}CO_2$ from the whole body CO_2 storage capacity ($PCO_2 \times$ weight, ml) (Clode et al, 1967).

4 may then be calculated.

This approach, first described by Marie Clode (1966), has two advantages over the use of R alone. First, movement of CO_2 into stores may be taken into account; secondly, the CO_2 balance equation above yields a quantitative estimate of the excess CO_2, which is more closely related to lactic acid production than R alone. This value for CO_2 produced in excess of aerobic CO_2 is converted into a molar quantity, which is equivalent to lactic acid. By using the probable distribution of lactate in body water, the change in blood lactate may be estimated to within ± 1 mM/L (Clode and Campbell, 1969). The use of the equation will be illustrated using the examples of the previous chapter. The data required are $\dot{V}CO_2$, $\dot{V}O_2$, change in $P_{\bar{v}}CO_2$ from beginning to end of the study, duration of study, and body weight.

Example 1   Male, weight 85 kg (p. 132)

Power Output kpm/min	$\dot{V}CO_2$ ml/min	$\dot{V}O_2$ ml/min	$P_{\bar{v}}CO_2$ before mm Hg	$P_{\bar{v}}CO_2$ at end mm Hg	duration min
800	2000	2080	65 (400 kpm/min)	70	5

The components of the CO_2 balance are as follows:

1. Total CO_2 output $= \dot{V}CO_2 \times$ time
$$= 2000 \times 5$$
$$= 10{,}000 \text{ ml}$$

2. CO_2 from aerobic metabolism $= \dot{V}O_2 \times$ aerobic R.Q. $\times$ time
$$= 2080 \times 0.9 \times 5$$
$$= 9360 \text{ ml}$$

3. CO_2 storage $= \pm$ change in $P_{\bar{v}}CO_2 \times$ body weight
$$= (70 - 65) \times 85$$
$$= +425 \text{ ml}$$

4. CO_2 from lactic acid $= 10,000 - 9360 + 425$
$$= 1065 \text{ ml}$$
$$= 48 \text{ mM}$$

This is equivalent to the production of 48 mM lactic acid. Because lactic acid distributes in body water (approximately 60 per cent body weight), and blood consists of 80 per cent water, this will be equivalent to a rise in blood lactate of about 48.6 BW $\times$ 0.8 mM/L or $\dfrac{48}{0.5 \times 85}$ mM/L. This rise -1.1 mM/L $-$ is not excessive at this power output.

Example 2   Female, weight 75 kg (p. 135)

Power Output kpm/min	$\dot{V}CO_2$ ml/min	$\dot{V}O_2$ ml/min	$P_{\bar{v}}CO_2$ before mm Hg	$P_{\bar{v}}CO_2$ at end mm Hg	duration min
400	1340	1120	60 (200 kpm/min)	65	6

The CO_2 balance constructed for this patient is as follows:

$$1340 \times 6 = (1120 \times 0.9 \times 6) + (5 \times 75) + CO_2 \text{ (lactic)}$$

$$CO_2 \text{ (lactic)} = 8040 - 6048 + 375$$

$$= 2367 \text{ ml}$$

$$= 106 \text{ mM}$$

$$\text{Blood lactate increase} = \frac{106}{0.5 \times 75} \text{ mM/L}$$

$$= 2.8 \text{ mM/L}$$

This increase is excessive for the power output.

Example 3   Female, weight 51 kg (p. 136)

Power Output kpm/min	$\dot{V}CO_2$ ml/min	$\dot{V}O_2$ ml/min	$P_{\bar{v}}CO_2$ before mm Hg	$P_{\bar{v}}CO_2$ at end mm Hg	duration min
300	1060	940	72 (150 kpm/min)	83	5

The CO_2 balance reads as follows:

$$1060 \times 5 = (940 \times 0.9 \times 5) + (11 \times 51) + CO_2 \text{ (lactic)}$$

$$
\begin{aligned}
CO_2 \text{ (lactic)} &= 5300 - 4230 + 561 \\
&= 1631 \text{ ml} \\
&= 73 \text{ mM}
\end{aligned}
$$

Change in blood lactate $= 2.9$ mM/L

These three examples, the same patients used in the previous chapters, serve to emphasize the advantages of this approach in obtaining a quantitative indirect estimate of blood lactate changes. Although different values for the respiratory exchange ratio indicate differences in anaerobic metabolism, the CO_2 balance quantifies the differences by using the absolute levels of CO_2 in excess of its aerobic production and by allowing for the CO_2 which is produced but not excreted.

The method also has the advantage of being applicable in real time. Blood analysis of lactate is time consuming and, for most laboratories, expensive, unless many analyses are done at the same time. For this reason, the result is delayed, whereas with the CO_2 balance technique results are available at once.

Having demonstrated the analytical value of using excess CO_2 in the measurement of lactate production, the physiological implications should also be stressed. An increase in CO_2 production leads to an increase in the demand on ventilation; disproportionate increase in ventilation in relation to O_2 intake, appearing during an exercise test, usually indicates that a power output has been reached which cannot be met completely from aerobic metabolism (Examples 1 and 2, Chap. 9).

References

Clode, M.: CO_2 balance during exercise. J. Physiol. *184*:49–50, 1966.

Clode, M., and Campbell, E. J. M.: The relationship between gas exchange and changes in blood lactate concentrations during exercise. Clin. Sci. 37:263–272, 1969.

Clode, M., Clark, T. J. H. and Campbell, E. J. M.: The immediate CO_2 storage capacity of the body during exercise. Clin. Sci. 32:161–165, 1967.

Issekutz, B., Jr., Birkhead, N. C. and Rodahl, K.: Use of respiratory quotients in assessment of aerobic work capacity. J. Appl. Physiol. 17:47–50, 1962.

Naimark, A., Wasserman, K. and McIlroy, M. B.: Continuous measurement of ventilatory exchange ratio during exercise. J. Appl. Physiol. 19:644–652, 1964.

Chapter Twelve

INTERPRETATION – FURTHER EXAMPLES

This chapter will allow the reader to interpret data obtained in several examples, which will serve also to emphasize the type of information obtained from exercise tests. For each example we suggest that data from each test (Stage 1, Stage 2, and Stage 3) be analyzed separately; in this way the additional information gained from more complex data can be appreciated readily. The reader may prefer to construct graphs from the data, similar to those used in the preceding chapter; some normal standards and a four-quadrant diagram are given in Appendix 4. A brief interpretation follows each set of data, with comments regarding points of interest.

EXAMPLE 1

Patient: M. G., female, age 46
Height: 163 cm; Weight: 47 kg; L.B.M.: 40 kg
Vital Capacity: 2.75 L; FEV_1: 2.15 L; FEV_1/VC: 78%
Hemoglobin: 15.7 g/100 ml

STAGE 1 PROGRESSIVE MULTISTAGE TEST

W kpm/min	0	100	200	300
f_c beats/min	82	112	132	148
$\dot{V}_E$ L/min		15	18	30
V_T ml		610	610	680
$\dot{V}O_2$ ml/min		480	600	710
$\dot{V}CO_2$ ml/min		410	570	780

STAGE 2   STEADY STATE TEST

W	kpm/min	0	200
$\dot{V}O_2$	ml/min	203	605
$\dot{V}CO_2$	ml/min	160	557
R		0.79	0.92
f_c	/min	90	135
$\dot{V}_E$	L/min	9.4	24.0
f_b	/min	27	38
V_T	ml	351	630
P_ECO_2	mm Hg	15	21
$P_{ET}CO_2$	mm Hg	31	29
$P_{\bar{v}}CO_2$	mm Hg	44	52
mins			6

STAGE 3   TEST

W	kpm/min	0	200
P_aCO_2	mm Hg	33.0	31.0
V_D/V_T	ratio	.30	.23
$\dot{Q}_t$	L/min	2.9	5.5
V_s	ml	32	41
P_aO_2	mm Hg	90	99
$P_{A\text{-}a}O_2$	mm Hg	16	14
S_aO_2		.96	.97
$\dot{Q}_{va}/\dot{Q}_t$	%	2.6	1.4
pH		7.34	7.31
HCO_3	mM	17.5	15.0
La	mM	.64	3.0

Spirometry shows values which are within normal limits for patient's size.

The Stage 1 test showed a reduced maximum power output. This was due in part to her small size, but even taking this into account, the maximum power output was only 60 per cent of that expected, and $\dot{V}O_2$ max was less than 20 ml/kg. The cardiac frequency was elevated at all power outputs, and although the value during maximal exercise was not at the maximal level predicted for her age, extrapolation of the submaximal values shows that had she accomplished a further workload, a maximal cardiac frequency would have been found. Thus she was close to a cardiovascular limitation.

EXAMPLE 2   159

Ventilation was normal when related to power output but increased for the levels of $\dot{V}O_2$ and $\dot{V}CO_2$; a disproportionate increase in $\dot{V}_E$ occurred at the highest power output, due in part to an increase in $\dot{V}CO_2$. Although $\dot{V}_E$ is high, there was still plenty of ventilation reserve in that the ventilation at the maximal power output was only 40 per cent of the predicted maximal voluntary ventilation.

The Stage 2 results showed a high cardiac frequency, increased ventilation, high frequency of breathing, and low tidal volume. The mixed venous PCO_2 was low, so alveolar hyperventilation must have been present. However, it is impossible to fit normal values for cardiac output to the data; assuming the highest value for V_D/V_T compatible with airway dead space alone (0.3; high due to the low V_T), arterial PCO_2 is 30 mm Hg, cardiac output 5 liters per minute, and stroke volume only 38 ml. This solution would be compatible with the low end tidal PCO_2. The CO_2 output is high, and a CO_2 balance indicates an increase in lactate of 2 mM/L.

The Stage 3 results confirmed the low arterial PCO_2, normal V_D/V_T ratio, and reduced cardiac output and stroke volume. Although pulmonary gas exchange was normal (normal V_D/V_T, $P_{A-a}O_2$, and $\dot{Q}_{va}/\dot{Q}_t$), lactate accumulation has occurred, indicating an abnormal degree of anaerobic metabolism for this metabolic demand; this is consistent with a cardiovascular impairment leading to inadequate O_2 delivery.

Comments

In this patient, referred for assessment of dyspnea of gradually increasing severity since mitral valvotomy five years previously, the Stage 1 results suggested a cardiovascular limitation with low stroke volume, and anaerobic metabolism. The Stage 2 results confirmed this and suggested that cardiac output was very low. The Stage 3 results added little to the Stage 2 data. Some other points are pertinent in this patient: it is important to take body size into account when analyzing exercise data; it is an advantage to relate variables to $\dot{V}O_2$ and $\dot{V}CO_2$ rather than to power output; and a low tidal volume is commonly seen in patients with left-sided cardiac and pulmonary vascular disease.

EXAMPLE 2

Patient: O. G., male, age 26
Height: 173 cm; Weight: 140 kg; L.B.M.: 82 kg
Vital Capacity: 5.0 L; FEV_1: 3.44 L; FEV_1/VC: 69%
Hemoglobin: 15.4 g/100 ml

STAGE 1   PROGRESSIVE MULTISTAGE TEST

W kpm/min	0	200	300	400	500	600	700	800	90
f_c beats/min	75	120	132	141	150	161	173	179	18
$\dot{V}_E$ L/min		26	32	45	57	62	83	95	11
V_T ml		1230	1300	1410	1520	1620	1790	2160	230

EXAMPLE 2   161

STAGE 2   STEADY STATE TEST

W	kpm/min	0	300	600
$\dot{V}_{O_2}$	ml/min	310	1159	1850
$\dot{V}_{CO_2}$	ml/min	250	1031	1585
R		0.80	0.85	0.86
f_c	/min	72	135	162
$\dot{V}_E$	L/min	10.8	33	56
f_b	/min	15	25	38
V_T	ml	720	1350	1460
$P_E CO_2$	mm Hg	20	27	25
$P_{ET} CO_2$	mm Hg	30	32	29
$P_{\bar{v}} CO_2$	mm Hg	42	52	54
mins			6	6

STAGE 3 TEST

W	kpm/min	0	300	600
$P_a CO_2$	mm Hg	34	34	32
V_D/V_T	ratio	.33	.17	.19
$\dot{Q}_t$	L/min	7.0	12.8	15.7
V_s	ml	100	95	97
$P_a O_2$	mm Hg	80	83	85
$P_{A\text{-}a} O_2$	mm Hg	25	20	25
$S_a O_2$		.95	.95	.96
$\dot{Q}_{va}/\dot{Q}_t$	%	13	3	3
pH		7.40	7.38	7.34
HCO_3^-	mM	20	19	17
La	mM	0.8	1.2	2.8

Six months later:

Weight: 108 kg; VC: 5.24 L; FEV_1: 4.15 L; FEV_1/VC: 72%

STAGE 1   TEST

W kpm/min	0	400	500	600	700	800	900	1000	1100
f_c beats/min	72	112	123	131	143	151	161	172	182
$\dot{V}_E$ L/min		29	33	41	51	56	71	94	106
V_T ml		1090	1400	1550	1700	1850	1950	2220	2520

EXAMPLE 2   163

The anthropometry results show a severe degree of obesity, body fat being 40 per cent.

Spirometry is essentially normal with slight reductions in vital capacity, FEV_1 and FEV_1/VC ratio.

The Stage 1 results show that, allowing for the severe obesity, the maximal power output is only slightly reduced. Cardiac frequency is at the upper limit of normal and reaches a value close to the maximum heart rate predicted by age. Ventilation is high at all power outputs and reaches a value close to the maximal voluntary ventilation (120 liters per minute). Thus both the ventilatory and the cardiovascular systems appear to be reaching maximal adaptation combining to limit performance.

The Stage 2 results reveal a cardiac frequency which is high for the oxygen intake. Ventilation is also increased, shown by the low values for P_ECO_2. The mixed venous PCO_2 is also low, indicating that the increase in ventilation is due to an increase in alveolar ventilation, at least in part. The mixed venous to mixed expired PCO_2 difference is consistent with normal values for cardiac output and V_D/V_T ratio. A CO_2 balance suggests that lactate accumulation did not occur.

The Stage 3 results confirm alveolar hyperventilation with low P_aCO_2, and normal V_D/V_T ratio, cardiac output, and stroke volume. The arterial PO_2 is slightly reduced, with a widened alveolar arterial PO_2 difference; this improves during exercise when venous admixture ratio falls to normal values. The blood lactate has increased to an extent which is normal for the oxygen intake.

Comments

The Stage 1 results identified the limiting factors and showed a virtually normal cardiovascular response with hyperventilation. The Stage 2 and 3 results mainly confirmed these findings and, although documenting the changes more precisely, added little to the assessment. The CO_2 balance technique underestimated lactate accumulation; the reason for this may be the utilization of free fatty acids as a fuel source, with a lower value for the muscle respiratory quotient than that assumed for the purposes of the calculation.

The patient was retested after six months, at which time his weight had fallen to 108 kg and his exercise symptoms had improved considerably; improvements occurred in the spirometric measurements and in the maximum power output. Cardiac frequency and ventilation were less at all power outputs, and at maximum power output the cardiac frequency was similar to that recorded in the previous test. Ventilation, although close to the previous maximal value, was now only 73 per cent of the predicted maximal voluntary ventilation (145 L/min). The pattern of breathing had also improved.

EXAMPLE 3

Patient: M. C., male, age 36
Height: 178 cm; Weight: 65 kg; L.B.M.: 59 kg
Vital Capacity: 3.8 L; FEV$_1$: 3.0 L; FEV$_1$/VC: 79%
Hemoglobin: 13.5 g/100 ml

STAGE 1 PROGRESSIVE MULTISTAGE TEST

W kpm/min	0	100	200	300	400	500	600
f$_c$ beats/min	72	88	120	135	150	171	180
$\dot{V}_E$ L/min		19	20	24	30	35	55
V$_T$ ml		1300	1430	1550	1590	1680	1750

STAGE 2 STEADY STATE TEST

W	kpm/min	0	200	400
$\dot{V}O_2$	ml/min	220	725	992
$\dot{V}CO_2$	ml/min	190	710	1080
R		0.88	.98	1.09
f$_c$	/min	76	130	168
$\dot{V}_E$	L/min	8.6	26	42
f$_b$	/min	14	18	25
V$_T$	ml	600	1450	1700
P$_E$CO$_2$	mm Hg	20	24.0	22.0
P$_{ET}$CO$_2$	mm Hg	34	43	40
P$_{\bar{v}}$CO$_2$	mm Hg	56.0	67.0	80.5
mins			6	5

EXAMPLE 3   **165**

STAGE 3   TEST

W	kpm/min	0	200	400
P_aCO_2	mm Hg	40	40	38
V_D/V_T	ratio	0.4	.35	.38
$\dot{Q}_t$	L/min	3.2	6.3	7.7
V_s	ml	42	48	46
P_aO_2	mm Hg	80	90	85
$P_{A\text{-}a}O_2$	mm Hg	22	17	28
S_aO_2	%	.95	.95	.94
$\dot{Q}_{va}/\dot{Q}_t$		3	1	1
pH		7.38	7.32	7.27
HCO_3^-	mM	22	20	17
La	mM	.8	2.0	4.5

Spirometry is within normal limits.

Stage 1 test shows reduced maximal power output equivalent to an oxygen uptake of 1.5 liters, reduced to at least 60 per cent of the predicted value. The cardiac frequency is high at all levels and reaches the maximal heart rate predicted for his age. Ventilation is high at all workloads and increases at the highest levels. The pattern of breathing is normal, and the maximal voluntary ventilation is not reached.

The Stage 2 results confirm the increased cardiac frequency for a given oxygen intake and the increased ventilation. The mixed expired PCO_2 is low, and the gross elevation in mixed venous PCO_2 suggests that the low P_ECO_2 cannot be due to alveolar overventilation alone. It is impossible to give normal values for either the V_D/V_T ratio or cardiac output in order to fit the results; at the highest normal level for V_D/V_T (0.22), arterial PCO_2 will be 31 mm Hg; the calculated venoarterial content difference is nearly 20 volumes per 100 ml, which, when converted to oxygen content, exceeds the blood oxygen capacity ($1.3 \times Hb = 17$). Thus the V_D/V_T ratio must be increased in addition to cardiac output being low. The CO_2 balance shows an increase in lactate concentration of 1.3 mM/L during the first stage and 2 mM/L during the second stage of the study.

The Stage 3 results show that the V_D/V_T ratio is increased and cardiac output low with a very low stroke volume. The arterial PO_2 is normal; although the alveolar to arterial PO_2 difference is increased, this is accounted for by a high alveolar PO_2 and a wide arteriovenous oxygen content difference; venous admixture is normal. There is a fall in arterial pH, which is consistent with the increase in lactate concentration.

Comments

In this patient, who was investigated because of dyspnea and a systolic cardiac murmur, the Stage 1 results identified a reduced maximum power output due to a grossly reduced cardiac reserve and low stroke volume. Stage 2 results increased our information by demonstrating that in addition to cardiac output being low the V_D/V_T ratio was high. The Stage 3 results quantified these abnormalities but added little other information. Other points brought up in the analysis and interpretation of the data are the effect of reduced Hb on the calculation of the venoarterial CO_2 content difference, and the effect of a wide arteriovenous O_2 difference on the interpretation of the A-a Po_2 difference. Subsequent cardiac catheterization confirmed a low cardiac output with severe mitral incompetence.

EXAMPLE 4

Patient: G. R., male, age 61
Height: 178 cm; Weight: 65 kg; L.B.M.: 60 kg
Vital Capacity: 3.3 L; FEV$_1$: 1.1 L; FEV$_1$/VC: 33%
Hemoglobin: 14.8 g/100 ml

STAGE 1   PROGRESSIVE MULTISTAGE TEST

W kpm/min	0	100	200	300	400
f_c beats/min	95	105	112	120	130
$\dot{V}_E$ L/min		20	22	30	38
V_T ml		930	1150	1290	1310

STAGE 2   STEADY STATE TEST

W	kpm/min	0	250
$\dot{V}o_2$	ml/min	290	855
$\dot{V}co_2$	ml/min	288	830
R		1.00	0.97
f_c	/min	90	120
$\dot{V}_E$	L/min	15.5	40.1
f_b	/min	20	29
V_T	ml	780	1370
$P_E co_2$	mm Hg	16	18
$P_{ET} co_2$	mm Hg	34	43
$P_{\bar{v}} co_2$	mm Hg	44	58
mins			5

EXAMPLE 4   167

STAGE 3 TEST

W	kpm/min	0	250
P_aCO_2	mm Hg	32	41.5
V_D/V_T	ratio	.43	.48
$\dot{Q}_t$	L/min	5	11
V_s	ml	56	92
P_aO_2	mm Hg	83	47.5
$P_{A-a}O_2$	mm Hg	35.5	62.0
S_aO_2		.96	.82
$\dot{Q}_{va}/\dot{Q}_t$	%	14	35
pH		7.48	7.38
HCO_3^-	mM	25	23
La	mM	1.0	2.5

Spirometry shows severe airway obstruction.

The Stage 1 test results show a severe reduction in the maximal power output (about 50 per cent of the predicted average). The ventilatory response is slightly higher than normal and reaches a level at which further increases are limited by the reduced ventilatory capacity. The estimated maximal voluntary ventilation is 38 liters per minute (1.1×35). The frequency of breathing is low, but at the highest level of work an increase occurs; the tidal volume is well maintained considering the reduction in FEV_1, but when the frequency of breathing is increased at the maximal level, there is a fall in tidal volume. Although cardiac frequency is above the average normal value, it does not reach a level close to the maximum predicted for his age.

The Stage 2 test results yield similar quantitative information to the Stage 1 test. The cardiac frequency is high for the level of oxygen uptake but within the normal range. Ventilation is high for the CO_2 output, as shown by the reduced P_ECO_2. The mixed venous PCO_2 is normal. Testing the data with the four-quadrant diagram will show that the results are not compatible with a normal V_D/V_T ratio and cardiac output. Because the cardiac frequency is within normal limits, and the ventilatory capacity limited the maximum power output in the Stage 1 test, it is likely that cardiac output is normal and thus that the V_D/V_T ratio is elevated. P_aco_2 may be normal or high, although a normal value is suggested by the normal end tidal PCO_2. The respiratory exchange ratio is high, indicating a high CO_2 output for this level of oxygen uptake; however, because mixed venous PCO_2 has increased, we may conclude that the high CO_2 output is not due to the washing out of CO_2 from body stores.

A CO_2 balance calculation shows a change in lactic acid level of 2 mM/L, which is higher than would normally be expected at this level of oxygen uptake.

The Stage 3 test results show that the arterial P_{CO_2} is low at rest and normal during exercise; the V_D/V_T ratio is high, but cardiac output and stroke volume are normal. The arterial P_{O_2} is low at rest and falls markedly during exercise, with an increase in the alveolar-arterial difference and a fall in arterial O_2 saturation. The venous admixture ratio increases. The blood lactate level shows an increase similar to that predicted from the Stage 2 results and appears to be secondary to arterial hypoxemia.

Note that a correction must be applied to the venoarterial content difference derived from the P_{CO_2} difference because of arterial O_2 desaturation, which is not detected in the bloodless test. However, this correction amounts to only 0.8 ml/100 ml, which does not affect the qualitative Stage 2 interpretation.

Comments

The Stage 1 results demonstrated the severity of the functional impairment and identified the limiting factor to be reduced ventilatory capacity, which was compromised by hyperventilation. The Stage 2 results showed that underventilation was not present and that cardiac output was probably normal; however, the severity of the pulmonary gas exchange abnormality, with a gross O_2 transfer defect, was revealed only by the Stage 3 results, which also confirmed that the cardiac response was normal. This patient had long-standing chronic airway obstruction. Other pulmonary function tests were compatible with the diagnosis of severe pulmonary emphysema—increased lung volumes, lowered carbon monoxide transfer factor, and reduced pulmonary elastic recoil. A severe gas exchange disturbance was associated with an increase in the ventilation, which encroached on the reduced ventilatory capacity and resulted in a severe reduction in effort tolerance.

EXAMPLE 5

Patient: G. S., male, age 57
Height: 175 cm; Weight: 85 kg; L.B. M.: 68 kg
Vital Capacity: 2.6 L; FEV_1: 0.90 L; FEV_1/VC: 35%
Hemoglobin: 16.5 g/100 ml

EXAMPLE 5   169

STAGE 1   PROGRESSIVE MULTISTAGE TEST

W kpm/min	0	100	200	300	400	500	600
f_c beats/min	100	112	120	128	135	145	152
$\dot{V}_E$ L/min		12	15	18	23	29	34
V_T ml		700	750	835	1020	1405	1250

STAGE 2   STEADY STATE TEST

W	kpm/min	0	200	400
$\dot{V}_{O_2}$	ml/min	254	1080	1350
$\dot{V}_{CO_2}$	ml/min	216	900	1430
R		0.85	0.87	1.05
f_c	/min	85	130	150
$\dot{V}_E$	L/min	7.8	23	31
f_b	/min	18	19.5	19.5
V_T	ml	430	1170	1580
P_ECO_2	mm Hg	24	34	40
$P_{ET}CO_2$	mm Hg	48	53	58
$P_{\bar{v}}CO_2$	mm Hg	66	86	97
mins			6	7

STAGE 3 TEST

W	kpm/min	0	200	400
P_aCO_2	mm Hg	58	60.5	63
V_D/V_T	ratio	.42	.39	.33
$\dot{Q}_t$	L/min	8.4	11	14
V_s	ml	100	77	93
P_aO_2	mm Hg	58	62	64
$P_{A-a}O_2$	mm Hg	22	16	24
S_aO_2		.86	.87	.87
$\dot{Q}_{va}/\dot{Q}_t$	%	20	12	14
pH		7.36	7.32	7.28
HCO_3^-	mM	31	30	29
La	mM	0.7	1.4	2.4

Spirometry shows severe airway obstruction, together with some reduction in vital capacity. Other pulmonary function tests confirmed the severe obstructive impairment (total lung capacity was normal and residual volume increased).

The Stage 1 results reveal a moderately reduced exercise performance (60 to 70 per cent of the predicted value). Cardiac frequency is somewhat high at all power outputs but at the maximal power output is lower than the maximal heart rate predicted from age. Ventilation is low at all levels of power output and reaches a value close to the predicted maximal voluntary ventilation (32 L/min).

The Stage 2 results confirm that cardiac frequency is high at both 200 and 400 kpm/min; this is due in part to the high $\dot{V}O_2$ at both levels, but even when this is allowed for, cardiac frequency is at the upper limit of normal. Ventilation is low for the $\dot{V}CO_2$, and P_ECO_2 is elevated to 40 mm Hg; the mixed venous PCO_2 is also very high. These results indicate that P_aCO_2 must be high: if $\dot{Q}_t$ were normal, P_aCO_2 would be at least 58 mm Hg at 400 kpm/min. The increased value for CO_2 output together with the increase in mixed venous PCO_2 at the higher workload indicates lactate accumulation, and a CO_2 balance shows an increase of 1.7 mM/L during this workload.

The Stage 3 results confirm the high arterial PCO_2 both at rest and during exercise, with increased V_D/V_T ratio and normal cardiac output and stroke volume. Arterial PO_2 is low at rest but increases during exercise, with little change in the alveolar-arterial PO_2 difference. The calculated venous admixture falls with exercise. The fall in arterial pH is due partly to the increase in PCO_2 and partly to a small increase in lactate.

Comments

The Stage 1 results demonstrated a relatively well maintained exercise tolerance, underventilation, and limitation due to reduced ventilatory capacity. The Stage 2 results suggested that severe underventilation occurred during exercise. The Stage 3 results confirmed this quantitatively and also demonstrated a normal cardiac output. Although a severe pulmonary gas exchange abnormality is present, this improves with exercise, presumably due to better distribution of ventilation:perfusion relationships.

This patient had severe chronic bronchitis with longstanding airway obstruction and abnormal gas exchange. It should be noted that compared with Example 4, in whom the ventilatory impairment was less severe but effort intolerance more marked, the underventilation allows a relatively high power output to be achieved before a ventilatory limit is reached, while the increase in arterial PO_2 with exercise allowed oxygen delivery to be maintained.

In analyzing the measurement of cardiac frequency and ventilation, this case emphasizes again the importance of relating measurements to O_2 intake and CO_2 output rather than power output alone.

Example 6   171

EXAMPLE 6

Patient: J. K., male, age 16
Height: 175 cm; Weight: 72 kg; L.B.M.: 68 kg
Vital Capacity: 3.33 L; FEV$_1$ 2.75 L; FEV$_1$/VC: 83%
Hemoglobin: 16.9 g/100 ml

STAGE 1   PROGRESSIVE MULTISTAGE TEST

W kpm/min	0	100	200	300	400	500	600	700	800
f_c beats/min	110	125	138	145	152	162	176	182	191
$\dot{V}_E$ L/min		22	27	31	35	47	79	93	99
V_T ml		610	650	730	930	1110	1330	1600	1510

STAGE 2   STEADY STATE TEST

W	kpm/min	0	300	500
$\dot{V}_{O_2}$	ml/min	252	816	1240
$\dot{V}_{CO_2}$	ml/min	190	860	1300
R		0.76	1.05	1.05
f_c	/min	120	160	180
$\dot{V}_E$	L/min	9	34	74
f_b	/min	24	31	56
V_T	ml	370	1090	1320
P_{ECO_2}	mm Hg	18	21	15
P_{ETCO_2}	mm Hg	31	29	24
$P_{\bar{v}CO_2}$	mm Hg	46	55	61
mins			5	6

STAGE 3 TEST

W	kpm/min	0	300	500
P_{aCO_2}	mm Hg	32	30	26
V_D/V_T	ratio	.26	.23	.36
$\dot{Q}_t$	L/min	2.7	7.2	8.4
V_s	ml	23	45	47
P_{aO_2}	mm Hg	76	70	61
P_{A-aO_2}	mm Hg	32	48	62
S_{aO_2}		.95	.94	.91
$\dot{Q}_{va}/\dot{Q}_t$	%	7	8	10
pH		7.39	7.38	7.37
HCO_3^-	mM	18.8	17.5	14.6
La	mM	0.8	2.2	4.8

Spirometry – there is a moderate reduction in the ventilatory capacity of nonobstructive type.

The Stage 1 results show that the maximum power output is reduced to about 80 per cent of the average value for patient's age. Cardiac frequency was increased at all levels and reached a value close to that expected for his age. Ventilation was also increased at the higher power outputs and at the highest level was close to the maximal voluntary ventilation (96 L/min). Tidal volume is reduced at all levels. Thus in addition to showing a ventilatory impairment with low tidal volume, a cardiovascular abnormality is suggested by the high cardiac frequency.

The Stage 2 results showed a gross increase in ventilation with very low $P_E CO_2$. The pattern of breathing was that of a high frequency with low tidal volume. The mixed venous PCO_2 was normal. It is impossible to fit normal values for V_D/V_T ratio and cardiac output to the data; the low end tidal PCO_2 suggests that there was marked alveolar hyperventilation, implying a low cardiac output in addition to an increased V_D/V_T; and a CO_2 balance indicates an increase in lactate of about 2 mM/L at each of the two workloads.

The Stage 3 results reveal a marked alveolar hyperventilation, increased V_D/V_T ratio, and low cardiac output and stroke volume. In addition, the arterial PO_2 was low at rest and fell with exercise, with a very large alveolar to arterial PO_2 difference and increasing venous admixture. There was a fall in bicarbonate and pH, which coincided with the increase in blood lactate.

This patient showed a gross increase in the alveolar-arterial PO_2 difference and thus provides an opportunity to examine the calculations made using the "3-compartment lung model" approach, in which arterial PCO_2 is assumed to be equal to the ideal alveolar PCO_2 in the calculation of alveolar PO_2. Arterial PCO_2 was 26 mm Hg at 500 kpm/min: using the calculated value for venous admixture (10 per cent) and the measured mixed venous PCO_2, we may calculate the extent to which the arterial PCO_2 is higher than the ideal alveolar PCO_2 (Riley et al, 1951):

$$0.9 \text{ (ideal } P_A CO_2) + 0.1 \text{ (61)} = 26$$

$$\text{Ideal } P_A CO_2 = 22.2 \text{ mm Hg}$$

Using this value instead of $P_a CO_2$, V_D/V_T is 0.28 (compared with 0.36), $P_A O_2$ is 127 mm Hg (instead of 123), and A-a PO_2 is 66 mm Hg (instead of 62). The differences between these figures are not great and do not lead to important errors of interpretation; however, the "second approximation" calculation employed above may be used in cases where doubt exists.

EXAMPLE 6   173

Comments

In this patient with allergic alveolitis, the true situation of the severe gas exchange disturbance, hypoxemia, and low cardiac output was not shown up clearly in the Stage 1 or 2 tests. This case also demonstrates the drawbacks to using the prediction of the normal expected response; prior to his illness he had been an extremely active youth, and on being tested two months later, when his pulmonary reaction had settled (see below), his performance was better than the predicted average, which shows that the degree of impairment was severe when first seen. Maximum power output increased from 800 kpm/min to 1300 kpm/min in two months and a year later reached 1600 kpm/min. Comparison of the results on the two occasions shows the importance of retesting. It will be noted also that the data obtained from Stage 1 and 2 tests were adequate to indicate the degree of improvement. A final point of interest is that the pathology was not impairing pulmonary gas exchange alone but also was embarrassing the circulation, presumably by causing pulmonary hypertension.

Two months later:
Weight: 80 kg; L.B.M.: 72 kg
Vital Capacity: 4.75 L; FEV_1: 4.3 L; FEV_1/VC: 90%
Hemoglobin: 15.5 g/100 ml

STAGE 1   TEST°

W kpm/min	0	600	700	800	900	1000	1100	1200	1300
f_c beats/min	95	134	138	145	156	159	174	180	191
$\dot{V}_E$ L/min		36	38	48	51	52	70	87	101
V_T ml		1710	1900	2180	2130	2700	2500	3000	2900

° Data at 100–500 kpm/min deleted.

STAGE 2   STEADY STATE TEST

W	kpm/min	0	400	800
$\dot{V}_{O_2}$	ml/min	260	1270	2130
$\dot{V}_{CO_2}$	ml/min	210	1080	2120
R		0.8	0.85	0.99
f_c	/min	100	135	174
$\dot{V}_E$	L/min	8.8	32	59
f_b	/min	15	22	26
V_T	ml	590	1440	2270
$P_E CO_2$	mm Hg	21	30	31
$P_{ET} CO_2$	mm Hg	34	39	37
$P_{\bar{v}} CO_2$	mm Hg	43	57	67
mins			5.5	6

EXAMPLE 7   175

STAGE 3 TEST

W	kpm/min	0	400	800
P_aCO_2	mm Hg	36	38	36
V_D/V_T	ratio	.31	.17	.11
$\dot{Q}_t$	L/min	7	12.4	17.7
V_s	ml	70	92	101
P_aO_2	mm Hg	80	88	84
$P_{A-a}O_2$	mm Hg	15	13	26
S_aO_2		.96	.96	.96
$\dot{Q}_{va}/\dot{Q}_t$	%	7	2	3
pH		7.40	7.38	7.35
HCO_3^-	mM	24	22	19
La	mM	0.6	1.5	4.2

EXAMPLE 7

Patient: A. K., male, age 41
Height: 175 cm; Weight: 71 kg; L.B.M.: 62 kg
Vital Capacity: 3.8 L; FEV_1: 3.2 L; FEV_1/VC: 84%
Hemoglobin: 14 g/100 ml

STAGE 1   PROGRESSIVE MULTISTAGE TEST

W kpm/min	0	100	200	300	400	500	600
f_c beats/min	90	95	100	102	105	112	120
$\dot{V}_E$ L/min		42	32	38	33	38	40
V_T ml		670	650	660	810	1040	1200

Spirometry was normal.

Stage 1 test. The patient, who was referred for assessment of shortness of breath, stopped exercising at a power output well below the expected normal value, and the highest level was graded "exhausting." Neither the cardiac frequency nor ventilation reached values considered to be limiting. Cardiac frequency was above normal at low power outputs but approached the normal range at higher levels. The striking abnormality was the increased ventilation at low power outputs, together with a large variation: the hyperventilation was less at higher power outputs, and the relative increase in ventilation normally found at power outputs close to maximum was not seen. This suggested that anaerobic metabolism did not occur, which was confirmed by a measurement of blood lactate taken shortly after the cessation of exercise that was only 2.5 mM/L.

Because of apparent apprehension the test was repeated a week later, with almost identical results being obtained.

This pattern of response is typical of psychogenic dyspnea, which confirmed the clinical impression: the patient showed clinical evidence of an anxiety reaction, together with episodes of dizziness and tingling that generally occurred at times of stress. The exercise test results excluded pulmonary hypertension and significant cardiac or pulmonary disease, allowing the physician to reassure the patient and pursue an expectant course of management with sedation. This clinical problem is not uncommon and deserves to be diagnosed promptly, before undue attention reinforces the patient's anxiety (Burns and Howell, 1969).

EXAMPLE 8

Patient: D. E., male, age 38
Height: 170 cm; Weight: 75 kg; L. B. M.: 60 kg
Vital Capaicity: 4.8 L; FEV_1: 4.0 L; FEV_1/VC: 83%
Hemoglobin: 15 g/100 ml

STAGE 1   PROGRESSIVE MULTISTAGE TEST

W kpm/min	0	100	200	300	400	500	600	700
f_c beats/min	66	79	85	96	103	106	121	130
$\dot{V}_E$ L/min		16	16	25	30	36	38	47
V_T ml		740	740	980	990	1050	1210	1280
BP	$\dfrac{130}{100}$		$\dfrac{145}{100}$		$\dfrac{150}{100}$		$\dfrac{155}{100}$	

STAGE 2   STEADY STATE TEST

W	kpm/min	0	200	400
$\dot{V}O_2$	ml/min		905	1130
$\dot{V}CO_2$	ml/min		685	945
R			0.75	0.83
f_c	/min	70	90	105
$\dot{V}_E$	L/min		20.0	25.5
f_b	/min		21	25
V_T	ml		950	1020
P_ECO_2	mm Hg		30	32
$P_{ET}CO_2$	mm Hg		38	39
$P_{\bar{v}}CO_2$	mm Hg		51	56
mins			5	6

EXAMPLE 9   177

Spirometry — normal.

The Stage 1 results show a reduced maximum power output, equivalent to a $\dot{V}_{O_2}$ max of 1.5 to 1.8 L/min. Cardiac frequency at the maximum level was well below that expected for his age (185 beats/min) and ventilation also was not limiting. Both cardiac frequency and ventilation were within normal limits at all workloads. Tidal volume was slightly low due to a high breathing frequency. Blood pressure was normal.

The results do not show any abnormality other than the low maximum power output and suggest poor motivation.

The Stage 2 results are all within normal limits and compatible with normal cardiac output and stroke volume, normal V_D/V_T ratio, and absence of significant lactic acid production.

He was referred for severe fatigue and effort intolerance, which had been present for two years following an aortic valve replacement.

The results enabled the patient to be strongly reassured and a positive approach taken to his lack of motivation and poor occupational work performance, which was due to a neurosis associated with the noise generated by the aortic valve replacement and to a wish for a disability pension.

The Stage 1 results were sufficient to answer the clinical questions, although the addition of the Stage 2 results was helpful in establishing that cardiac output was normal.

EXAMPLE 9

Patient: S. P., female, age 24
Height: 158 cm; Weight: 53 kg; L.B.M.: 40 kg
Vital Capacity: 3.2 L; FEV_1: 2.7 L; FEV_1/VC: 84%
Hemoglobin: 13 g/100 ml

STAGE 1 PROGRESSIVE MULTISTAGE TEST

W kpm/min	0	100	200	300	400	500	600*
$\dot{V}_{O_2}$ ml/min		214	335	617	740	960	1050
$\dot{V}_{CO_2}$ ml/min		290	290	470	650	940	1060
f_c beats/min	90	112	120	134	150	168	178
$\dot{V}_E$ L/min		13	15	18	23	29	
V_T ml		550	720	750	750	990	

*Power output not completed (30 sec)

STAGE 2   STEADY STATE TEST

W	kpm/min	0	300
$\dot{V}O_2$	ml/min	150	940
$\dot{V}CO_2$	ml/min	140	860
R		.93	.91
f_c	/min	96	149
$\dot{V}_E$	L/min	5.5	24.6
f_b	/min	14	27
V_T	ml	390	910
P_ECO_2	mm Hg	24.3	30.2
$P_{ET}CO_2$	mm Hg	38	38
$P_{\bar{v}}CO_2$	mm Hg	46	60

STAGE 3 TEST

W	kpm/min	0	300
P_aCO_2	mm Hg	37	38
V_D/V_T	ratio	.12	.14
$\dot{Q}_t$	L/min	3.5	9.6
V_s	ml	36	64
P_aO_2	mm Hg	92	97
$P_{A-a}O_2$	mm Hg	18	11
S_aO_2		.96	.97
$\dot{Q}_{va}/\dot{Q}_t$	%	4	2.5
pH		7.38	7.33
HCO_3^-	mM	21.6	20.3
La	mM	1.0	2.6

Spirometry is normal.

The *Stage 1 results* show a reduction in maximum power output: note that body fat is 26 per cent of body weight and that at a lean body mass of 40 kg the maximum predicted O_2 uptake is about 1.8 L/min. Measured $\dot{V}O_2$ max was 1050 ml/min. The cardiac frequency at the maximum power output is close to the predicted maximum of 194 beats/min and is elevated at all submaximal power outputs. Ventilation, on the other hand, is normal at all power outputs. The electrocardiograph was normal.

The *Stage 2 results* are all normal apart from a high cardiac frequency and are compatible with normal cardiac output and V_D/V_T ratio and normal lactate production.

Example 10   179

The *Stage 3 results* confirm normal cardiac output and pulmonary gas exchange variables.

In this patient, a nurse referred for investigation of severe effort intolerance associated with fatigue, the Stage 1 results suggest a low stroke volume, but the absence of an increase in CO_2 output and in ventilation do not support a cardiovascular limitation sufficient to cause lactate production. The Stage 2 results are compatible with normal cardiac output and V_D/V_T ratio, and this is confirmed by the Stage 3 results.

The Stage 2 results were required to establish that cardiac output was normal.

The results, together with the clinical assessment, were compatible with the diagnosis of vasoregulatory asthenia (Holmgren et al, 1957).

EXAMPLE 10

Patient: S. G., male, age 54
Height: 170 cm; Weight: 88 kg; L.B.M.: 72 kg
Vital Capacity: 5.5 L; FEV_1: 4.3 L; FEV_1/VC: 79%
Hemoglobin: 16 g/100 ml

STAGE 1   PROGRESSIVE MULTISTAGE TEST

W	0	200	300	400	500	600	700	800	900	1000
$\dot{V}O_2$		950	1130	1230	1450	1540	1740	1990	2220	2210
$\dot{V}CO_2$		820	920	1010	1200	1400	1580	2010	2380	2600
f_c	62	94	98	105	106	108	114	118	124	130
V_E		27	32	34	40	46	52	60	72	88
V_T		1130	1280	1330	1560	1850	2180	2370	2380	2890
BP	112/80		160/100		170/100		180/100		190/100	

Spirometry was normal.

The resting electrocardiograph was normal.

Stage 1 test. The maximum power output was 1000 kpm/min, and the patient stopped because of leg fatigue and dyspnea. Although this is within the normal range for adult men of his age, with a maximum O_2 intake of 2220 ml/min, it represents only 25.2 ml/kg; thus for his size this maximum value is in the lower normal range.

The cardiac frequency was low at all power outputs and at maximum was considerably lower than the maximum for his age (175 beats/min). Ventilation was normal at the lower power outputs but high at the submaximal levels; however, the ventilation at maximum was well below the predicted maximum ventilatory capacity. This behavior, which was associated with an increase in CO_2 output, suggests that lactic acid production occurred, a conclusion confirmed later by the blood lactate measured during the second minute of recovery, which was 6.5 mM/L. This in turn suggested that O_2 transport mechanisms had reached limiting values.

The resting electrocardiograph showed changes compatible with an old anterior infarction, but no ST segment changes occurred during or after exercise.

In view of the low cardiac frequency, stroke volume must be normal. However, the inability of cardiac frequency to increase to normal maximal values appeared to be a factor limiting maximal exercise.

This patient, who had suffered a myocardial infarction a year previously, was referred for exercise testing prior to enrollment in an activity program. From the results of the test a training level was chosen equivalent to an O_2 intake of 1.8 L/min or 6 METS (multiples of resting O_2 intake), and at which cardiac frequency was 110 to 120 beats/min. Further studies were not required.

CONCLUSION

Our aim in the latter part of the book has been to illustrate how the information obtained from simple exercise techniques may be applied to a variety of clinical situations in order to answer some of the questions raised in the first chapter.

The full value of exercise testing in clinical medicine comes from an understanding of the integrated series of processes that deliver O_2 and remove CO_2. The clinician may then appreciate the significance of the findings in his patients, and exercise testing becomes an extension of the clinical history and examination. In addition to adding detail and precision to the assessment of exercise-related symptoms, factors may come to light which contribute to the functional disturbance but which were undetected clinically. Finally, exercise testing allows the clinician to advise patients regarding everyday activities: often the results may be used to reassure patients that serious heart or lung disease is not present.

Increasing familiarity with exercise tests leads to extensive use, which in turn not only improves their value to the clinician but also broadens the range of clinical conditions in which he finds them of help. The growing and laudable concern with improved standards of fitness in the general population will encourage the use of exercise testing to prescribe safe but effective exercise regimes and to provide evidence of improvement. The publicity surrounding the "coronary-prone" individual has also resulted in wider use of exercise testing in diagnosis, prescription, and assessment of exercise programs. Also the realization that physical fitness improves the quality of life in ways over and above the possible prevention of heart attacks will lead to a growing demand on physicians for advice regarding appropriate exercise regimes. This demand will require physicians to be well informed regarding exercise testing and fitness and also to have access to testing facilities. In the narrower medical context, exercise testing is almost certain to be increasingly applied in the assessment of drugs acting on the cardiovascular and respiratory systems.

An increasing use of exercise testing will, we believe, further emphasize the value of simple exercise tests, particularly for screening and to assess progress. It is likely that techniques similar to the Stage 1 procedure described in this book will allow physicians to perform tests in their offices. Other techniques, simpler to administer and perform, will also be valuable, particularly for follow-up and motivation of patients taking part in exercise programs. Progress has been made towards tests that require no special equipment and which may be self-administered by the general population.

During the next few years, new techniques will be developed and evaluated for application to a number of clinical situations. Noninvasive measures of myocardial function and cardiac output may prove to be valuable additions to routine exercise testing in cardiac patients. Biochemical and histochemical techniques will become further refined to allow muscle biopsy to be more widely applied; from this we may gain important information regarding changes at the tissue level that have a bearing on fitness and the effects of training. Light may be shed also on conditions such as vasoregulatory asthenia, in which the factors leading to impaired function are presently obscure. Electrophysiological techniques may identify conditions in which the functional abnormality is at the level of the motor unit.

Whatever additional information is obtained from these techniques, we can be certain that the basis for informative exercise tests will always be the classical physiology of the processes which supply O_2 to the tissues and remove CO_2 from them. The series of linked mechanisms which discharge these functions can already be comprehensively studied using the techniques we have described.

Inherent in our approach is the use of interrelationships between mechanisms for analytical reasons as well as to obtain a physiological description of the system under stress. The principles of testing at several power outputs with a systematic examination of the mechanisms as they adapt to increasing demands will remain central to any technique developed in the future, and we are confident that the analytical framework will also stand the test of time. We hope that this book has restated these principles and, by describing some simple techniques, will have opened the door to their wider application.

References

Burns, B. H., and Howell, J. B. L.: Disproportionately severe breathlessness in chronic bronchitis. Quart. J. Med. 38:277–294, 1969.

Holmgren, A., Jonsson, B., Levander, M., Linderholm, H., Sjöstrand, T., and Ström, G.: Low physical working capacity in suspected heart cases due to inadequate adjustment of peripheral blood flow (vasoregulatory asthenia). Acta Med. Scand. 158:413–436, 1957.

Riley, R. L., Cournand, A., and Donald, K. W.: Analysis of factors affecting partial pressure of oxygen and carbon dioxide in gas and blood of lungs: Methods. J. Appl. Physiol. 4:102–120, 1951.

Appendix One

SYMBOLS

The convention established by Pappenheimer et al (1950) has been followed, with primary symbols (what is measured) and suffixes (where it is measured).

PRIMARY SYMBOLS

C = concentration in blood phase
D = diffusion
F = fractional concentration in dry gas phase
f = frequency
G = any gas
P = pressure in general, including partial pressure
$\dot{Q}$ = volume flow or blood per unit time, including cardiac output
S = oxygen saturation of hemoglobin in per cent
T = time
V = gas volume in general
$\dot{V}$ = volume flow of gas per unit of time

PREFIXES AND SUFFIXES

1. Gas Phase
   A = alveolar
   B = barometric
   D = dead space
   E = expired
   I = inspired
   ET = end tidal (e.g., $P_{ET}CO_2$)
   T = tidal (e.g., V_T)

2. Blood Phase
   a = arterial
   c = capillary
   v = venous
   $\bar{v}$ = mixed venous
   c´= end capillary
   p = plasma
3. Miscellaneous Functions
   b = breathing (e.g., f_b)
   c = cardiac (e.g., f_c)
   s = stroke (e.g., V_s)
   t = total
   va = venous admixture

ABBREVIATIONS

ATPS = Ambient temperature, pressure, saturated with water vapor

BTPS = Body temperature (ambient), pressure, Saturated with water vapor

STPD = Standard temperature (0° C), pressure (760 mm Hg), Dry

Appendix Two

CALCULATION
OF RESULTS

The principles underlying calculations have been mentioned previously (p. 90). This section will enable you to carry out the calculations, given basic measurements, and will cover all the calculations needed in a steady state exercise test. A recording such as the one illustrated in Figures A-1 and A-2 will have been produced during the test (Chap. 4).

CONSTRUCTION OF CALIBRATION LINES
FOR CARBON DIOXIDE AND OXYGEN

The upper channel of the recorder covers the range of the three lowest calibrating CO_2 mixtures (which contain oxygen at a concentration similar to expired gas), and the lower channel records the higher concentrations of CO_2 required for measurements during rebreathing (these calibrating gases contain about 40 per cent oxygen). The deflections are identified and a line drawn (Fig. A-1) from which unknown CO_2 concentrations can be read (mixed expired, end tidal, and rebreathing P_{CO_2}). If the recorder is being used to measure mixed expired O_2 concentration, a similar calibration line is drawn (Fig. A-1).

MEASUREMENTS FROM COLLECTION OF
EXPIRED GAS (FIG. A–2)

1. Time Factor: the number of centimeters of recorder paper passing in one minute. Because the recorder speed control may not be

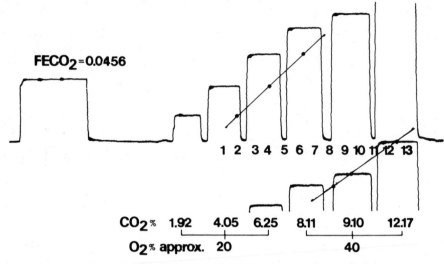

FECO$_2$=0.0456

1 2 3 4 5 6 7 8 9 10 11 12 13

CO$_2$% 1.92   4.05   6.25   8.11   9.10   12.17

O$_2$% approx.   20   40

TISSOT ANALYSIS + CALIBRATION OF CAPNOGRAPH

Figure A-1   Construction of calibration curve for CO$_2$ analyzer and analysis of CO$_2$ concentration in mixed expired gas.

accurate, the time factor should be measured using the time base, which is accurate.

2. Volume Factor: liters entering the Tissot spirometer or passing through the dry gas meter to produce 1 cm deflection. If the volume corresponding to one complete revolution of the potentiometer— that is, one complete sweep length (x, liters)—is known, division of that volume by the vertical deflection on the paper of a complete sweep (y, cm) produces the required value $\left(\dfrac{x}{y}, L/cm\right)$.

3. Time Measurement: centimeters of paper for the period of gas collection.

4. Volume Deflection: centimeters of paper measured vertically during the period of collection.

5. Cardiac Frequency Deflection: centimeters of paper, measured horizontally, corresponding to 5 ECG R-R intervals.

6. Breathing Frequency Deflection: number of breaths during collection period.

MEASUREMENTS FROM ANALYSIS OF GAS
(FIG. A-2)

1. F_ECO_2.   Fractional concentration of carbon dioxide in the mixed expired gas (top calibration line).

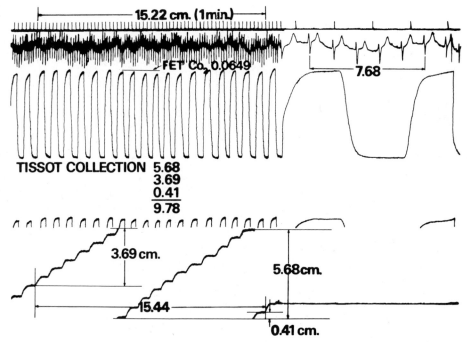

Figure A–2   Measurement of cardiac frequency, end tidal CO_2 concentration, and ventilation.

2. F_EO_2:   Fractional concentration of oxygen in mixed expired gas.
3. $F_{ET}CO_2$:   Fractional concentration of carbon dioxide at the mouthpiece at the end of expiration (using top calibration line), averaged for the period of collection.
4. $F_{\bar{v}}CO_2$:   Fractional concentration of carbon dioxide at the mouthpiece during a rebreathing equilibrium (Fig. A–3).

OTHER DATA REQUIRED

1. P_B.   Barometric Pressure.
2. T.   Temperature of mixed expired gas in the spirometer.
3. BTPS Correction.   Converts gas volume measured at a temperature (T) in atmospheric pressure and saturated with water vapor (ATPS) to the volume expressed at body temperature (37° C).

$$\text{BTPS} = \dot{V}_{\text{ATPS}} \times \frac{273 + 37}{273 + T} \quad \frac{P_B - PH_{H_2O,\ T}}{P_B - 47} \quad \textbf{(Table A–1)}$$

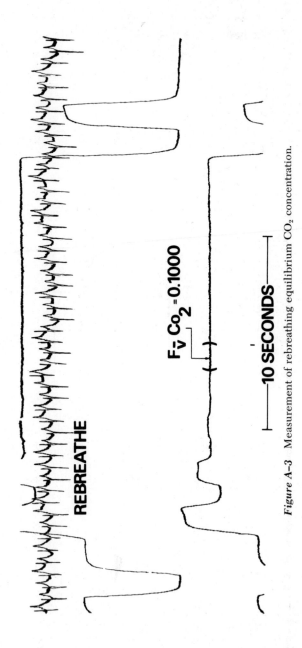

Figure A–3   Measurement of rebreathing equilibrium CO_2 concentration.

4. STPD   Converts the gas volume at ATPS to that at standard temperature (0° C) and pressure (760), dry.

$$\dot{V}_{STPD} = \dot{V}_{ATPS} \times \frac{273}{273 + T} \quad \frac{P_B - P_{H_2O,T}}{760} \quad \textbf{(Table A–2)}$$

5. Hb.   Hemoglobin concentration (grams/100 ml).

CALCULATION OF RESULTS

1. *Cardiac Frequency* (beats/min)

$$f_c = \frac{50 \times a}{e}$$

2. *Ventilation* (L/min)

$$\dot{V}_E \ (\text{BTPS}) = \frac{d \times b \times a \times \text{BTPS factor}}{c}$$

$$\dot{V}_E \ (\text{STPD}) = \frac{d \times b \times a \times \text{STPD factor}}{c}$$

3. *Breathing Frequency* (breaths/min)

$$f_b = \frac{f \times a}{c}$$

4. *Tidal Volume* (ml)

$$V_T = \frac{\dot{V}_E \ (\text{BTPS}) \times 100}{f_b}$$

5. *O$_2$ Intake, CO$_2$ Output* (ml/min)

$$\dot{V}_{CO_2} = F_E CO_2 \times \dot{V}_E, \text{STPD} \times 1000$$
$$\dot{V}_{O_2} = 1000 \ [(\dot{V}_I, \text{STPD} \times 0.2093) - (\dot{V}_E, \text{STPD} \times F_E O_2)]$$

where

$$\dot{V}_I, \text{STPD} = \dot{V}_E, \text{STPD} \times \left[\frac{1 - F_E O_2 - F_E CO_2}{0.7904} \right]$$

$$R = \frac{\dot{V}_{CO_2}}{\dot{V}_{O_2}}$$

6. CO_2 Pressures (mm Hg)

$$P_ECO_2 = F_ECO_2 \times (P_B - 47)$$

$$P_{ET}CO_2 = F_{ET}CO_2 \times (P_B - 47)$$

$$P_{bag}CO_2 = F_{\bar{v}}CO_2 \times (P_B - 47)$$

A correction factor is applied to this value to derive "true" mixed venous PCO_2 ($P_{\bar{v}}CO_2$), for the reasons outlined on page 60. $P_{\bar{v}}CO_2 = P_{bag}CO_2 - [(0.24\ P_{bag}CO_2) - 11\ mm\ Hg]$

7. Pulmonary Gas Exchange

$$V_D = \left[\frac{P_aCO_2 - P_ECO_2}{P_aCO_2} V_T \right] - \text{Instrumental Dead Space}$$

$$\dot{V}_A = \frac{\dot{V}CO_2 \times 0.863}{P_aCO_2}$$

$$P_AO_2 = [F_IO_2 \times (P_B - 47)] - P_aCO_2 \left(F_IO_2 + \frac{1 - F_IO}{R} \right)$$

(the alveolar air equation)

8. Estimation of Arterial Pco_2

If P_aCO_2 has not been measured, it can be predicted from $P_{ET}CO_2$ as follows (Robertson et al, 1974):

$$P_aCO_2 = P_{ET}CO_2 + 4.4 - 0.0023\ V_T + 0.03\ f_b - 0.09\ P_ECO_2$$

Or it may be calculated from P_ECO_2 using an average value for physiological dead space. In adult males, mean $V_D = 138.4 + 0.077\ V_T$ ml (Jones et al, 1966). For other subjects a value may be predicted from body size (Radford, 1954):

$$P_aCO_2 = P_ECO_2 \div \left(1 - \frac{V_D + V_{D\ app}}{V_T} \right)$$

where $V_{D\ app}$ is the dead space volume of the respiratory valve.

9. Cardiac Output

The arteriovenous content difference of carbon dioxide is first obtained by calculating the arterial and venous contents separately and subtracting one from the other.

$$\log_e CCO_2 = 0.396 \times \log_e PCO_2 + 2.4$$

$$CCO_2 = \text{antilog}(\log_e CCO_2) ml/100\ ml$$

The content difference is then corrected for the patient's hemoglobin and arterial O_2 saturation.

a. Correction if Hb concentration is not 15 g/100 ml:
$$C'_{\bar{v}\text{-}a}CO_2 = C_{\bar{v}\text{-}a}CO_2 - [(15 - Hb) \times 0.015 \times (P_{\bar{v}}CO_2 - P_aCO_2)]$$
b. Correction for S_aO_2:
$$C'_{\bar{v}\text{-}a}CO_2 = C_{\bar{v}\text{-}a}CO_2 - [(100 - S_aO_2) \times 0.064]$$
where $C'_{\bar{v}\text{-}a}CO_2$ is the "corrected" venoarterial content difference. The venoarterial CO_2 content difference may also be calculated by using McHardy's transformation of the CO_2 dissociation curve (the lower right quadrant of the four-quadrant diagram), which has been constructed for Hb 15 g/100 ml and S_aO_2 95 per cent: similar corrections are applied. For Hb the equation above is used; for S_aO_2 the following equation is used:

$$C'_{\bar{v}\text{-}a}CO_2 = C_{\bar{v}\text{-}a}CO_2 - [(95 - S_aO_2) \times 0.064]$$

$$\dot{Q}_t = \frac{\dot{V}CO_2}{C'_{\bar{v}\text{-}a}CO_2 \times 10} \ L/min$$

$$V_s = \frac{\dot{Q}_t \times 1000}{f_c} \ ml$$

Venous admixture ratio is calculated by converting PO_2 measurements to O_2 saturation, $S_{c'}O_2$ obtained from P_AO_2, and applying the following equation:

$$\frac{\dot{Q}_{va}}{\dot{Q}_t} = \frac{S_{c'}O_2 - S_aO_2}{S_{c'}O_2 - S_{\bar{v}}O_2} \times 100$$

where $S_{\bar{v}}O_2 = S_aO_2 - \dfrac{\dot{V}O_2 \times 10}{\dot{Q}_t \times Hb \times 1.34}$

EXAMPLE OF CALCULATION

Workload: 200 kpm/min (see Figs. A-1, A-2, and A-3)

Stage 2 Test Measurements

Barometric Pressure	745
Temperature	22°C
BTPS Factor	1.0921
Volume Factor	1.80
Time Factor	15.22
Cardiac Frequency Deflection	7.68
Volume Deflection	9.78
Time Deflection	15.44
Number of Breaths	18
$F_E CO_2$	0.0456
$F_E O_2$	0.1588
$F_{ET} CO_2$	0.0649
$F_{\bar{v}} CO_2$	0.1000

Calculations

$$f_c = \frac{50 \times 15.22}{7.68} = 99 \text{ beats/min}$$

$$\dot{V}_E \text{ (ATPS)} = \frac{9.78 \times 1.80 \times 15.22}{15.44} = 17.35 \text{ L/min}$$

$$\dot{V}_E \text{ (BTPS)} = 17.35 \times 1.0921 = 18.95 \text{ L/min}$$
$$\dot{V}_E \text{ (STPD)} = 17.35 \times 0.8829 = 15.32 \text{ L/min}$$
$$f_b = \frac{18 \times 15.22}{15.44} = 17.7 \text{ breaths/min}$$

$$V_T = \frac{18.948}{17.7} = 1070 \text{ ml}$$

$$\dot{V}CO_2 = 0.0456 \times 15.319 \times 1000 = 699 \text{ ml}$$
$$\dot{V}O_2 = 15.319 \left(\frac{0.2093 \times (1 - 0.1588 - 0.0456)}{0.7904} - 0.1588 \right) = 795 \text{ ml}$$

$$R = \frac{699}{794} = 0.88$$

$$P_E CO_2 = 0.0456 \times 698 = 32 \text{ mm Hg}$$
$$P_{ET} CO_2 = 0.0649 \times 698 = 45 \text{ mm Hg}$$
$$P_{bag} CO_2 = 0.1000 \times 698 = 68.9 \text{ mm Hg}$$
$$P_{\bar{v}} CO_2 = 68.9 - [(0.24 \times 68.9) - 11] = 63.1 \text{ mm Hg}$$

DERIVATION OF $\dot{Q}_t$ AND V_D/V_T FROM P_aCO_2 ESTIMATED FROM $P_{ET}CO_2$ OR MEASURED

Measurements

$P_{ET}CO_2 = 45$ mm Hg
$V_T = 1070$ ml
$f_b = 17.7$ breaths/min
$P_ECO_2 = 32$ mm Hg

Calculations

$P_aCO_2 = 45 + 4.4 - (.0023 \times 1070) + (0.03 \times 17.7) - (0.09 \times 32)$
$\qquad = 44.6$ mm Hg

$V_D = \left(\dfrac{44.6 - 32}{44.6} \times 1070 \right) - 60$
$\quad = 242$ ml

$V_D/V_T = \dfrac{242}{1070}$
$\qquad = 0.23$

$C_aCO_2 = $ antilog $[(\log_e 44.6 \times 0.396) + 2.4]$
$\qquad = $ antilog 3.90
$\qquad = 49.4$ ml/100 ml

$C_{\bar{v}}CO_2 = $ antilog $[(\log_e 63.1 \times 0.396) + 2.4]$
$\qquad\quad = 56.9\ 1$ ml/100 ml

(No corrections are required for Hb or S_aO_2.)

$\dot{Q}_t = \dfrac{699}{(56.9 - 49.4)} \times 10$

$\quad = 9.3$ L/min

$V_s = \dfrac{9300}{99}$

$\quad = 94$ ml

Additional Calculations Performed When P_aO_2 Is Measured

MEASUREMENTS

P_aCO_2 = 46 mm Hg
P_aO_2 = 85 mm Hg
pH = 7.40
S_aO_2 = 95.6%
Hb = 15 g/100 ml

CALCULATIONS

C_aO_2 = 0.956 (Hb × 1.38)
     = 19.8 ml/100 ml

$$P_AO_2 = [0.2093 \times (745 - 47)] - 46 \left(0.2093 + \frac{0.7904}{0.88}\right)$$

= 95.0 mm Hg

($Cc'O_2$ = 20 ml/100 ml)

$P_{A\text{-}a}O_2$ = 10 mm Hg

$$\dot{Q}_{va}/\dot{Q}_t = \frac{20.0 - 19.8}{20.0 - 12.4}$$

$$\left(\text{where } C_{\bar{v}}O_2 = C_aO_2 - \frac{\dot{V}O_2}{\dot{Q}_t}\right)$$

= 0.02 (2%)

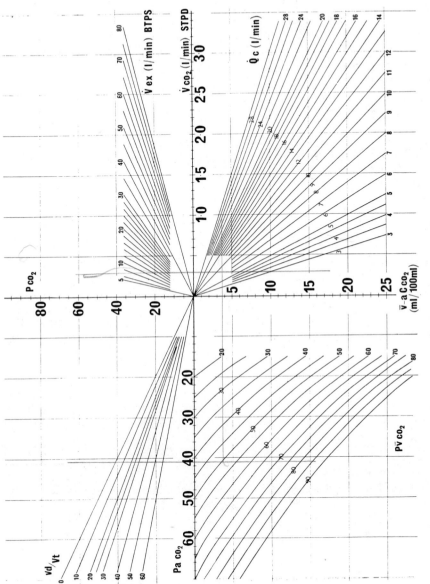

Figure A–4 Four-quadrant diagram (Chap. 10).

Appendix Three

CONVERSION FACTORS AND CONSTANTS

TABLE A–1 CONVERSION OF TRADITIONAL UNITS TO SI (SYSTÈME INTERNATIONALE) UNITS

INDEX	SYMBOL	TRADITIONAL UNITS	SI UNITS	CONVERSION FACTOR (F)[*]
Ventilation	$\dot{V}$	$l\ min^{-1}$ (L/min)	$l\ min^{-1}$	1
Pressure or tension	P	cmH_2O	kPa	0.098
		mm Hg (or torr)	kPa	0.133
Gas uptake	$\dot{n}$	$ml\ min^{-1}$ (ml/min)	$mmol\ min^{-1}$	22.4^{-1}[**]
Gas content in blood	C	$ml\ dl^{-1}$ (ml/100 ml)	$mmol\ l^{-1}$	2.24^{-1}[**]
Gas transfer factor	T	$ml\ min^{-1}\ torr^{-1}$ (ml/min/mm Hg)	$mmol\ min^{-1}kPa^{-1}$	0.335
Energy expenditure	–	calories	joules	4.18

[*]That is, $SI = TU \times F$.

[**]For O_2 and most other gases; for CO_2 the factor is 22.26^{-1}, or, in the case of CO_2 content in blood, 2.226^{-1}.

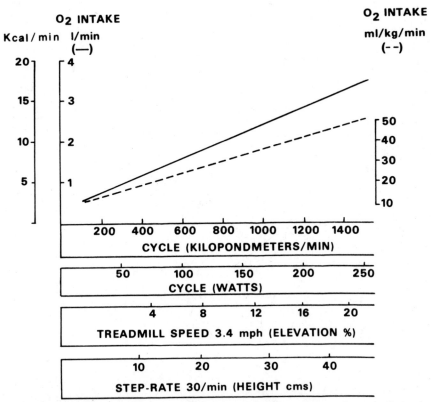

Figure A-5   Graph to convert power output generated in a variety of tests to O_2 intake and Kcal/min for a 70 kg man. For other weights use O_2 intake/kg/min for treadmill and step tests, which employ body lift.

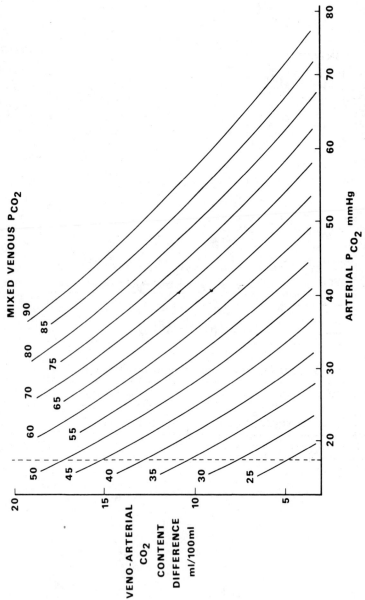

Figure A–6 Graph to convert mixed venous-arterial P$_{CO_2}$ difference to content difference (McHardy, 1967). Hb 15 g/100 ml, arterial O$_2$ saturation .95.

TABLE A-2 FACTORS TO CONVERT VOLUMES MEASURED AT ATPS TO BTPS AND STPD

	TEMPERATURE AT WHICH MEASURED					
	20°	21°	22°	23°	24°	25°
Water Vapor Pressure (mm Hg)	17.5	18.7	19.3	21.1	22.4	23.8
BTPS *Factor*	1.102	1.096	1.091	1.085	1.080	1.075
STPD Factors at P_B of						
740	.878	.874	.869	.864	.860	.855
742	.885	.881	.876	.871	.867	.862
744	.888	.883	.878	.874	.869	.864
746	.890	.886	.881	.876	.872	.867
748	.892	.888	.883	.879	.874	.869
750	.895	.890	.886	.881	.876	.872
752	.897	.893	.888	.883	.879	.874
754	.900	.895	.891	.886	.881	.876
756	.902	.898	.893	.888	.883	.879
758	.905	.900	.896	.891	.886	.881
760	.907	.902	.898	.893	.888	.883
762	.910	.905	.900	.896	.891	.886
764	.912	.907	.903	.898	.893	.888
766	.915	.910	.905	.900	.896	.891
768	.917	.912	.908	.903	.898	.893
770	.919	.915	.910	.905	.901	.896
772	.922	.917	.912	.908	.903	.898
774	.924	.920	.915	.910	.905	.901
776	.927	.922	.917	.912	.908	.903
778	.929	.924	.920	.915	.910	.905
780	.932	.927	.922	.917	.912	.908

TABLE A–3 ACTIVITY EQUIVALENTS

POWER OUTPUT KPM/MIN	WATTS	O₂ INTAKE L/MIN	METS*	ENERGY KCAL/MIN	WALK MPH	RUN MPH	CYCLE MPH	OCCUPATION	SPORT
300	50	0.9	4–5	5	3			Housework Clerical	Golf Bowls
600	100	1.5	7–8	8	4.5			Farming Mining Heavy Industry	Tennis Dancing Canoeing
900	150	2.1	8–10	11	5	5.5	12	Very heavy manual labor	Basketball Skiing
1200	200	2.8	12	14		7	16		Squash Cross-country skiing Hockey
1500	250	3.5	14	17		8	20		Competitive endurance sports
1800	300	4.2	16	20		10			rowing cross-country skiing
2100	350	5.0	18	24					running swimming

*METS = multiples of resting O₂ intake (3.5 to 4.0 ml O₂/kg/min)

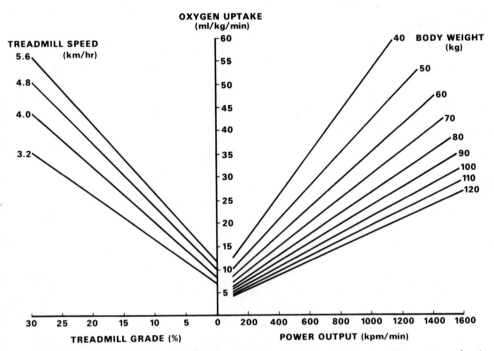

Figure A–5A   Graph comparing O_2 intake in a progressive exercise test (Stage I procedure) performed on a cycle ergometer and treadmill, obtained in a study of 6 healthy subjects.

The right-hand portion of the graph was obtained from measurements of O_2 intake at each power output in a Stage I test performed on a cycle ergometer. The left-hand portion was obtained from measurement of O_2 intake in treadmill tests performed at the 4 speeds shown, using progressive increments in elevation of 2.5 per cent each minute. (J. R. Wicks, unpublished observations, 1975.)

The graph enables data obtained in a Stage I test performed on a treadmill to be compared with data obtained with a cycle ergometer. The treadmill speed and elevation are converted into an equivalent power output by drawing a horizontal line to the isopleth for the subjects' weight in the right-hand graph. Data such as cardiac frequency and ventilation may then be compared with the values established using cycle ergometry. The graph may be used also to predict maximal O_2 intake from data obtained in both treadmill and cycle ergometer tests.

Appendix Four

NORMAL STANDARDS

PREDICTION OF MAXIMAL O_2 INTAKE ($\dot{V}O_2$ MAX)

In children aged 8 and above with normal body fat, $\dot{V}O_2$ max may be predicted by using a factor of 50 ml O_2/min/kg in males and 45 ml O_2/min/kg in females (Lange-Anderson et al, 1971).

$\dot{V}O_2$ max in adults gradually declines with age. The following equations predict $\dot{V}O_2$ max in healthy adults aged 20 years and above and are derived from data obtained in Europe, Scandinavia, and North America (Åstrand, P.-O., 1956; Åstrand, I, 1960; Lange-Anderson et al, 1971; and Shephard, 1969).

Males

$$\dot{V}O_2 \text{ max} = 4.2 - 0.032 \text{ age L/min (SD } \pm 0.4)$$
$$\dot{V}O_2 \text{ max} = 60 - 0.55 \text{ age ml/kg/min (SD } \pm 7.5)$$

Females

$$\dot{V}O_2 \text{ max} = 2.6 - 0.014 \text{ age L/min (SD } \pm 0.4)$$
$$\dot{V}O_2 \text{ max} = 48 - 0.37 \text{ age ml/kg/min (SD } \pm 7.0)$$

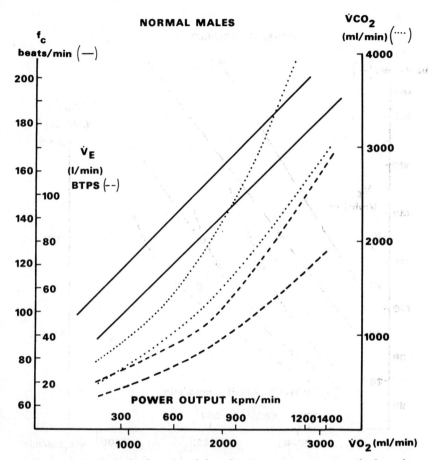

Figure A–7 Normal values for adult males, Stage 1 exercise test: the boundaries represent ± SD from the mean values at each power output.

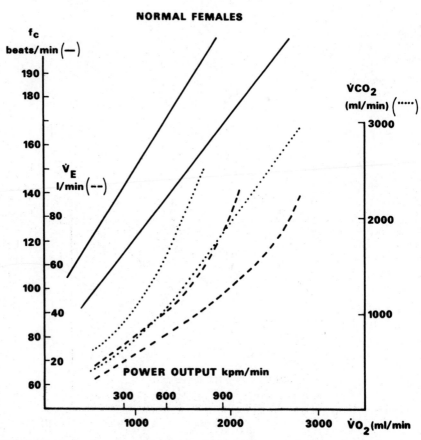

Figure A-8   Normal values for Stage 1 test, adult females: boundaries ± SD from mean.

TABLE A–4 GUIDE TO NORMAL VALUES: STAGE 2 AND 3 TESTS, MALES 20–60*

Variable	Symbol		Power Outputs				Variance or SD	Comments
			200 (33)	400 (66)	600 (100)	800 (133)		
Power Output	w kpm/min	(watts)	200 (33)	400 (66)	600 (100)	800 (133)	10%	
O_2 Intake	$\dot{V}O_2$	ml/min	800	1200	1600	2000	10%	
CO_2 Output	$\dot{V}CO_2$	ml/min	700	1150	1600	2100	10%	
Resp. Exchange Ratio	R		0.90	0.95	1.00	1.05	10%	
Cardiac Frequency	f_c	beats/min	95	110	125	140	12%	Relate to size.
Ventilation	V_E	L/min	20	32	42	58	15%	
Breathing Frequency	f_b	/min	18	20	20	24	15%	
Tidal Volume	V_T	ml	1100	1600	2100	2400	25%	Relate to FEV_1
Mixed expired PCO_2	P_ECO_2	mm Hg	30	31	32.5	31	3 mm Hg	
End Tidal PCO_2	$P_{ET}CO_2$	mm Hg	42	43	44	42	5 mm Hg	
Mixed Venous PCO_2	$P_{\bar{v}}CO_2$	mm Hg	60	63	66	70	5 mm Hg	
Arterial PCO_2	P_aCO_2	mm Hg	40	40	40	36	2 mm Hg	
Dead Space/Tidal Volume	V_D/V_T		.20	.18	.15	.12	.4	Relate to V_T. Corrected for instrumental V_D (60 ml).
Cardiac Output	$\dot{Q}_t$	L/min	9.0	12.5	14.0	16.0	2 L/min	
Stroke Volume	V_s	ml	95	110	115	115	10%	Relate to size.
Arterial PO_2	P_aO_2	mm Hg	90	92	92	92	4 mm Hg	
Alveolar-arterial PO_2 Diff.	$P_{A-a}O_2$	mm Hg	12	12	14	16	5 mm Hg	
Arterial O_2 Saturation	S_aO_2	%	.963	.965	.965	.960	.005	
Venous Admixture	$\dot{Q}_{va}/\dot{Q}_t$		4	3	3	3	1	
pH	pH		7.40	7.39	7.38	7.35	.02	
Bicarbonate	HCO_3^-	mM/L	24.0	23.5	23.0	21.5	2.0 mM/L	
Lactate	La	mM/L	1.0	1.5	2.0	3.5	2.0 mM/L	

*Average values representative of healthy nonsmoking males, average weight 80 kg. Figures rounded off and variances are also averaged.

TABLE A–5 GUIDE TO NORMAL VALUES: STAGE 2 AND 3 TESTS, FEMALES 20–50*

Variable	Symbol		Power Outputs			Variance or SD
Power Output	w kpm/min	(watts)	200 (33)	400 (66)	600 (100)	
O$_2$ Intake	$\dot{V}O_2$	ml/min	800	1200	1550	12%
CO$_2$ Output	$\dot{V}CO_2$	ml/min	720	1180	1630	12%
Resp. Exchange Ratio	R		.90	.98	1.05	10%
Cardiac Frequency	f_c	beats/min	108	130	155	12%
Ventilation	$\dot{V}_E$	L/min	22	33	48	25%
Breathing Frequency	f_b	/min	18	19	24	15%
Tidal Volume	V_T	ml	1200	1700	2000	25%
Mixed Expired Pco$_2$	P_ECO_2	mm Hg	28	30	29	3.5 mm Hg
End Tidal Pco$_2$	$P_{ET}CO_2$	mm Hg	40	40	39	5 mm Hg
Mixed Venous Pco$_2$	$P_{\bar{v}}CO_2$	mm Hg	56	61	65	5 mm Hg
Arterial Pco$_2$	P_aCO_2	mm Hg	38	36	35	3.5 mm Hg
Dead Space/Tidal Volume	V_D/V_T		.20	.13	.11	.04
Cardiac Output	$\dot{Q}_t$	L/min	9	11.5	14	2 L/min
Stroke Volume	V_s	ml	85	90	90	15 ml
Arterial Po$_2$	P_aO_2	mm Hg	92	91	92	6 mm Hg
Alveolar-arterial Po$_2$ Diff.	$P_{A-a}O_2$		14	17	22	4 mm Hg
Arterial O$_2$ Saturation	S_aO_2	%	.965	.965	.961	.010
Venous Admixture	$\dot{Q}_{va}/\dot{Q}_t$		3	3	3	1.5
pH	pH		7.40	7.4	7.36	.04
Bicarbonate	HCO_3^-	mM/L	22.5	22.0	20.0	3 mM/L
Lactate	La	mM/L	1.0	2.0	4.0	2 mM/L

*Average values representative of healthy nonsmoking women, average weight 60 kg.

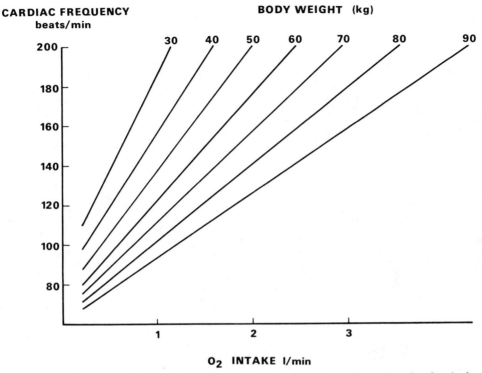

Figure A–9 Normal values for cardiac frequency in children and adults, related to body weight.

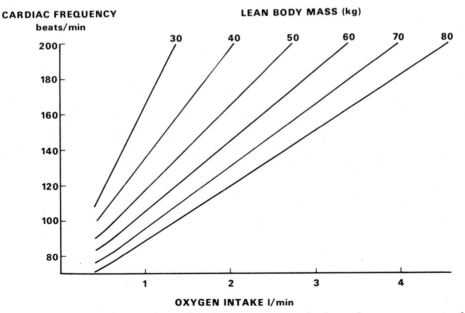

Figure A–10 Graph to predict cardiac frequency in normal subjects from measurements of lean body mass. Derived from data of Cotes et al (1973), Gadhoke and Jones (1969), and Godfrey et al (1971). Variance is approximately 10 per cent.

207

References

Åstrand, I.: Aerobic work capacity in men and women with special reference to age. Acta Physiol. Scand. Suppl. 196, 1960.

Åstrand, P.-P.: Human physical fitness, with special reference to sex and age. Physiol. Rev. 36:307–335, 1956.

Cotes, J. E., Berry, G., Burkinshaw, L., Davies, C. T. M., Hall, A. M., Jones, P. R. M. and Knibbs, A. V.: Cardiac frequency during submaximal exercise in young adults; relation to lean body mass, total body potassium and amount of leg muscle. Quart. J. Exp. Physiol. 58:239–250, 1973.

Gadhoke, S., and Jones, N. L.: The responses to exercise in boys aged 9 to 15. Clin. Sci. 37:789–801, 1969.

Godfrey, S., Davies, C. T. M., Wozniak, E. and Barnes, C. A.: Cardiorespiratory response to exercise in normal children. Clin. Sci. 40:419–431, 1971.

Jones, N. L., McHardy, G. J. R., Naimark, A. and Campbell, E. J. M.: Physiological dead space and alveolar-arterial gas pressure differences during exercise. Clin. Sci. 31:19–29, 1966.

Lange-Anderson, K., Shephard, R. J., Denolin, H., Varnauskas, E. and Masironi, R.: Fundamentals of exercise testing. World Health Organization, Geneva, 1971.

McHardy, G. J. R.: Relationship between the difference in pressure and content of carbon dioxide in arterial and venous blood. Clin. Sci. 32:299–309, 1967.

Pappenheimer, J. R., Comroe, J. H., Cournand, A., Ferguson, J. K. W., Filley G. F., Fowler, W. S., Gray, J. S., Helmholtz, H. F., Otis, A. B., Rahn, H. and Riley, R. L.: Standardization of definitions and symbols in respiratory physiology. Fed. Proc. 9:602, 1950.

Radford, E. P., Jr.: Ventilation standards for use in artificial respiration. J. Appl. Physiol. 7:451, 1955.

Robertson, D. G., Jones, N. L. and Kane, J. W.: Estimation of arterial P_{CO_2} from end tidal P_{CO_2} in exercising adults. In press, 1975.

Shephard, R. J.: Endurance fitness. Toronto, University of Toronto Press, 1969.

APPENDIX FIVE: GUIDE TO MANUFACTURERS

Manufacturer	Anemometer	Blood Gas Analyzer	CO₂ Analyzer	Chem. Gas Analyzer	Cycle Ergometer	Douglas Bags	Gas Meter	O₂ Analyzer (FAST)	O₂ Analyzer (SLOW)	Pneumotachograph	Recorder	Taps	Tissot Spirometer	Treadmill	Tubing	Valves
Automated Medical Systems Inc., Minneapolis, Minnesota 55420 U.S.A.			X					X								
Beckman Instrument, Inc., Palo Alto, California 94304 U.S.A.			X					X	X		X					
British Oxygen Company, London W6, England	X														X	
Gould Inc. Brush Div., Cleveland, Ohio 44114, U.S.A.											X					
Cardiopulmonary Instruments, Houston, Texas 77036 U.S.A.					X	X			X							
Collins, Warren, E., Inc., Braintree, Massachusetts 02184 U.S.A.					X	X						X	X		X	X
Corning Scientific Inst., Medfield, Massachusetts 02052 U.S.A.		X										X	X		X	X
Dargatz, A., Hamburg 1, Germany					X											
Devices Instruments Ltd., Welwyn, Garden City, England	X										X					
Dräger Werk, 24 Lüdeck Moislinger Allee 53–55 Germany		X		X												
Eschweiler & Co., Kiel, Germany		X		X	X											
Fleish, Lausanne, Switzerland										X						

Manufacturer	Anemometer	Blood Gas Analyzer	CO_2 Analyzer	Chem. Gas Analyzer	Cycle Ergometer	Douglas Bags	Gas Meter	O_2 Analyzer (FAST)	O_2 Analyzer (SLOW)	Pneumotachograph	Recorder	Taps	Tissot Spirometer	Treadmill	Tubing	Valves
Gallenkamp, London, E.C.2, England				X												
Gilson Medical Electronics Inc., Middleton, Wisconsin 53562 U.S.A.											X					
Grubb Parsons, Newcastle Upon Tyne N#6 2YB England																X
Hans Rudolph, Kansas City, Missouri 64114 U.S.A.											X	X				
Hewlett Packard—Vertek, Palo Alto, California U.S.A.											X	X				
Honeywell Inc., Denver, Colorado, U.S.A.												X				
Instrumentation Laboratories, Lexington, Massachusetts 02173 U.S.A.		X														
Instrumentation—Lode N.V., Groningen, Holland					X											
Leeds and Northrup, North Wales, Pa. 19454 U.S.A.									X							
Litton Medical Products, Inc., Elk Grove, Illinois 60001 U.S.A.					X						X					
Monark Crescent AB, Varberg, Sweden																
Narco, Houston, Texas, U.S.A.										X	X					
Ohio Medical Products, Madison, Wisconsin 53701 U.S.A.							X									
Parkinson Cowan Ltd., Stretford, Manchester, England								X								
Perkin Elmer, Pomona, California 91767 U.S.A.			X					X								
Quinton Instruments, Seattle, Washington 98199 U.S.A.		X			X									X		
Radiometer, Copenhagen NV, Denmark		X														
Scientific Research Instruments Co., Baltimore, Maryland 21207 U.S.A.		X	X		X			X	X		X					
Siemens-Elema, Solna 1, Postfack S-171 20 Sweden		X	X		X			X	X		X					
Servomex Controls Ltd., Crowborough, Sussex, England								X	X							
Statham-Godart, Bilthoven, Holland		X	X					X								
Varian Mat GMbH, Bremen, West Germany		X	X					X								
Westinghouse, Pittsburgh, Pennsylvania 15221 U.S.A.								X								
Zentralwerkstatt, Gottingen G.M.B.H., Gottingen, W. Germany				X												

Index

211